"Thank you, Millers, for putting in one convenient book everything we tell the clients at Sacramento County Drug Court, and more! You've created not only a sourcebook for people tired of 'white-knuckling' their way through recovery, but also for those of us providing treatment who know that brain repair is the essential first step to release anyone from any addiction."

—Carolyn Reuben, LAc, author of *Cleansing the Body, Mind, and Spirit*, and President, Community Addiction Recovery Association

"A courageous step forward from two pioneers in the substance abuse field who have worked long and hard to present this new technology with a great voice. This important work in the integration of alternative treatment modalities for chemical dependency is long overdue."

—Stan Stokes, Executive Director of Bridging the Gaps

"The Millers are exceptional communicators and educators in the addiction field. This book offers groundbreaking, life-saving information for anyone involved in recovery."

—Dr. James Braly, author of *Dr. Braly's Food Allergy and Nutrition Revolution*

"Addiction treatment works, but comprehensive (complementary) treatment works better! This book is a marvelous way to keep what you've got or to get what you need."

—Dr. Jay M. Holder, President, American College of Addictionology and Compulsive Disorders

"Merlene and David are far ahead of their time. They are among the first to finally change the way we treat addiction in this country."

—Tamea Sisco, DD, CAd

Other Books by Merlene Miller and David Miller

STAYING SOBER: A GUIDE FOR RELAPSE PREVENTION
Terence T. Gorski and Merlene Miller

LEARNING TO LIVE AGAIN: A GUIDE FOR RECOVERY
FROM CHEMICAL DEPENDENCY
Merlene Miller, Terence Gorski, and David Miller

OVERLOAD: ATTENTION DEFICIT DISORDER AND
THE ADDICTIVE BRAIN
David Miller and Kenneth Blum

REVERSING THE WEIGHT GAIN SPIRAL
Merlene Miller and David Miller

COUNSELING FOR RELAPSE PREVENTION
Terence Gorski and Merlene Miller

REVERSING THE REGRESSION SPIRAL
Merlene Miller and David Miller

HOW TO QUIT
Patrick Holford, David Miller, and James Braly

Staying Clean & Sober

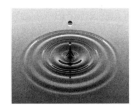

Complementary and Natural Strategies for Healing the Addicted Brain

Second Edition

**Merlene Miller, MA, and
David Miller, PhD**

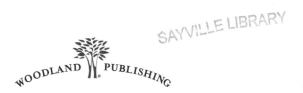

WOODLAND PUBLISHING

IN LOVING MEMORY OF DR. BEN

For permissions, ordering information, or bulk quantity discounts, contact: Woodland Publishing, Salt Lake City, UT

Visit our Web site: www.woodlandpublishing.com
Toll-free number (800) 777-BOOK

Note: The information in this book is for educational purposes only and is not recommended as a means of diagnosing or treating an illness. All matters concerning physical and mental health should be supervised by a health practitioner knowledgeable in treating that particular condition. Neither the publisher nor the authors directly or indirectly dispense medical advice, nor do they prescribe any remedies or assume any responsibility for those who choose to treat themselves.

ISBN 978-1-58054-124-4

Printed in the United States of America

Contents

Acknowledgments 7

1. The Search for Better Treatment 9

2. This Is Your Brain on Drugs;
   This Is Your Life on Drugs 19

3. The Pain of Ineffective Treatment and Relapse 49

4. Those Amazing Amino Acids 67

5. Intravenous Delivery of Mood-boosting Nutrients 91

6. This Is Your Brain on Food 103

7. Acupuncture, Auriculotherapy,
   and Cranial Electrical Stimulation 131

8. Brainwave Biofeedback (Neurofeedback) 141

9. Body Work 149

10. Essential Oil Therapy 157

11. Support People 165

12. Stress-Reducing Activities 173

13. Stress-Reducing Attitudes 197

14. Enriching Life 205

Appendix A: Putting It All Together 221

Appendix B: Chronic Abstinence Symptom Severity Scale 229

Appendix C: Deficiency Questionnaires 231

Resources 235

Notes 237

Suggested Reading 247

Index 249

Acknowledgments

WE HAVE HAD HELP IN WRITING THIS BOOK. And the message we share reflects the words and works of the dedicated people we consider part of our team. There is Stan Stokes and everyone at Bridging the Gaps in Winchester, Virginia, where comprehensive treatment is available; Jay Holder, who shared his knowledge and experience with addiction and specifically auriculotherapy; Jim Braly, who caught the vision for the future of IV amino acid therapy and supported our effort to make it a reality; Julia Ross, who felt for many years that she was a lone voice crying out for better treatment; Tamea Sisco, who took the risk to begin IV amino acid therapy at Excel Treatment Center before anyone had paved the way; Charles Gant for his pioneering work in alternative treatments for addiction; Karen Hurley, who has contributed so much to make recovery nutrients available to those who need them; Carol Cummings, Jeff Holbrook, and Dee Ogle, who have believed there is a better way and shared our dreams all along the way. The voices of these people are in this book and their work has led the way and guided us in our search for better treatment. We want to thank Debra and Matt Manka who have joined us in our journey. And thanks to Pat Smith who shares the vision. We also want to thank others who have shared with us information about their work and/or research: Joel Lubar, Kathy Sloan, Diana Guthrie, Richard Guthrie, Bill Hitt, Carolyn Reuben, and Kenneth Blum. We appreciate Jan Soan for all the help she gives us and for always being there when we need her. And thanks to Sue Sloan for what she does to help us and to make us look good. A very special thanks goes to our agent Stephanie von Hirschberg who has believed in the value of this book from the beginning and given us endless help and encouragement. We thank those at Woodland Publishing who have contributed to making this book a reality. Thanks to those who assisted in manuscript preparation: Teah Sloan, June Wright, Jan Sloan, Paul Kennard, and Jane Heywood. We are grateful to special friends who have supported us through our journey: Anne and Al Brady, Marilyn and John Shank, Terry and Hubert Rathbun, The Harrison Group, Dick and Jane Heywood, and Anne Barcus. Our wonderful family is always supportive and assists us in any way they can. Thanks to our parents, our sons, our daughters-in-law, and our grandchildren.

CHAPTER 1

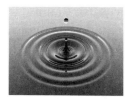

The Search for Better Treatment

WHEN I MET DAVID MILLER, he was an active alcoholic. I didn't recognize it because, as he has often said, I knew so little about alcoholism that I thought withdrawal was talking with a Southern accent. I thought he drank too much, but as I wasn't planning to marry him, I figured it was his business. But both those factors changed. What had been a close friendship developed into a deep love, and a life crisis caused him to make the decision to quit drinking. As far as I was concerned, the drinking problem was over and we were in love, so we got married.

His period of abstinence didn't last very long. And living with his drinking instead of observing it as an outsider was more of a problem than I knew how to deal with. I had four children from a previous marriage, and ultimately I felt I had to ask him to choose between us and his drinking. He chose us and began attending Alcoholics Anonymous. But his decision to stop drinking was just the beginning of our struggles. I thought that if he weren't drinking everything would be fine. I didn't realize that there are symptoms of addiction that emerge with abstinence that can make life nearly as uncomfortable as the drinking (many authorities now think these symptoms precede and contribute to addiction in the first place).

Without alcohol, David was moody, stress sensitive, and irritable. He was highly sensitive to noise (and all of my children are hearing impaired, resulting in a noisier than usual environment); and he sometimes found family life almost unbearable. He often withdrew from the rest of us, leaving me feeling depressed and rejected. Sometimes I thought it had been easier to live with him when he was drinking.

Despite this, I respected his effort to maintain sobriety even when I could see it was extremely difficult for him. I tried to be supportive, and he tried to give as much to the marriage as he was able. But sometimes the internal turmoil became so unbearable that he drank. For three years, he struggled to maintain sobriety (and periodically slipped) before he was able to maintain ongoing abstinence. He now has thirty-four years of continuous recovery.

David's years of sobriety are due somewhat to what we learned together about managing what we later called chronic abstinence symptoms of addiction. In all the meetings we attended, all the counseling we received, and all the reading we did, no one told us it would be so difficult. No one told us that these symptoms are frequently part of recovery. And no one told us what to do about them because, quite frankly, no one really knew.

We learned by trial and error to cope with David's symptoms. For instance, we noticed that the symptoms were worse on Saturdays. Why? As we looked at what was different we found a number of culprits. He slept later on Saturdays, thus ate later. In fact, he would often get up and go to his AA sponsor's house without eating. There he would drink coffee, eat donuts, and smoke cigarettes. And when he came home, he would find me vacuuming, the kids playing music, the phone ringing, and general chaos reigning. His only way of coping was to leave, which I resented. So when he did come back, even if things had settled down, I was usually not in a loving, supportive mood.

Eventually, because our desire to make our marriage better was so strong, we began to search for answers to the problems linked to David's fight with abstinence. Some of the steps we took were very simple. I began taking a glass of orange juice to him before he got out of bed to raise his blood sugar (and, though I didn't realize it at the time, to temporarily alter his brain chemistry). He started eating breakfast before he went to see his sponsor and refrained from the donuts and limited the coffee. Almost immediately, he was amazed at how different he felt. When he came home he was in a better mood, and I tried to reduce the typical noise and clamor. David made more of an effort to stick around and contribute to the Saturday needs of the family. But if things did become too stressful I tried to understand his need to get away for a time.

Gradually, David and I found other ways to help him maintain a more comfortable sobriety. We found ways to reduce noise levels in the home. We discovered that you can't just work at recovery. You have to play, too. We found that there must be creative and enjoyable activities to replace the void left by the absence of alcohol. What we were doing, but didn't realize at the time, was finding ways to alter the chemicals in the brain that help us feel good, the chemicals related to addiction: endorphins, enkephalins, serotonin, dopamine, and GABA.

Because of our efforts, we were not only able to hold our marriage together, but we also built a stronger relationship by working together to figure out how to live in sobriety. The point of this story is that long-term, lasting sobriety is difficult. It is not just a matter of willpower and self-discipline. It is not just a choice to stop using and go on with your life. What we came to understand was that addiction is a physiologically and biochemically linked condition and that there are physiological and biochemical symptoms that can't be ignored. We realized that when recovering addicts relapse it is usually not because they don't want to stay sober. It's because they don't know how.

What we learned by our own trial and error, and a lot of heartache, we wanted to share with other people in recovery. We determined to help others find alternatives to relapse and to the pain that often accompanies abstinence. To do that, we began looking for better and better ways to smooth out the road to recovery.

After a few years of ongoing recovery, David went back to school and became an addiction counselor. He was fortunate to work with Terry Gorski, who was also interested in relapse prevention. Terry was looking at what he called post-acute withdrawal, a group of symptoms he had found often accompanied abstinence. It was a relief to have a name for the symptoms David experienced and to realize that he was not alone. These symptoms were common in sobriety.

Together, Terry, David, and I wrote a book called *Learning to Live Again: A Guide to Recovery from Alcoholism* (later revised and called *Learning to Live Again: A Guide to Recovery from Chemical Dependency*). In this book we were able to share what we had learned about the road to recovery and how to make it smoother. And it was exciting to realize that other people could benefit from what we had learned the hard way.

Later, Terry and I wrote a book called *Staying Sober: A Guide to Relapse Prevention*. This book has been used widely in the addiction field since 1986. The reason for its wide acceptance is that people who read the book began learning for the first time about symptoms that make recovery difficult. They realize that they are not crazy or hopeless if they have these symptoms or if they relapse. What a relief.

In *Staying Sober* we say that post-acute withdrawal symptoms are due to damage to the nervous system from drug use and will go away as the brain and body heal. But what began to trouble David after a time was that for many people the symptoms never go away. They had never gone away for him. He had just learned how to cope with them, and after more than ten years of sobriety, these effects could still make him very uncomfortable.

Eventually, David and I had our own treatment program, and clients told us they still suffered from symptoms after many years of sobriety. Because we specialized in relapse prevention, most of the people we saw struggled with the symptoms and with periodic relapse. We realized that for some people recovery is not a road to walk but a mountain to climb. We developed our own strategy of relapse prevention and applied it to a variety of conditions, including food addiction. We wrote a book, *Reversing the Weight Gain Spiral*, about preventing relapse by compulsive overeaters.

As we taught clients about post-acute withdrawal symptoms, many of them told us that they had experienced the symptoms *before* they started drinking or using drugs (or overeating). They had the symptoms as long as they could remember. And they told us that these symptoms were the reason they started drinking or using drugs in the first place as self-medication for their discomfort.

David became convinced that what we were calling post-acute withdrawal, in many cases, was not really withdrawal but the return of symptoms that had been relieved by using addictive substances. He was especially sure of this in relation to the symptoms of heightened sensitivity to noise and lights and even touch. He began to learn more about this symptom, often called stimulus augmentation, or sometimes hyper-augmentation or hypersensitivity. His interest was further heightened because he had been plagued with this condition since he was a child.

David found that most chronic relapsers experienced stimulus augmentation. He discovered that people with attention deficit hyperactivity disorder (ADHD) frequently have this symptom and that people with ADHD often have alcohol and drug problems. He was ultimately diagnosed with attention deficit disorder himself and later, with the scientist Kenneth Blum, wrote the book *Overload: Attention Deficit Disorder and the Addictive Brain.* Through further research, David also discovered that many people in recovery from addiction have undiagnosed ADHD. As he continued his study, he found that there are other related disorders that predispose people to addiction, among them Tourette's syndrome, obsessive-compulsive disorder, depression, and conduct disorder. All these conditions are neurological and biochemical, meaning they are related to chemical imbalances in the brain. The more David and I analyzed the research related to addiction, the more aware we became of the gap between what is known about addiction and what is being done about it. As scientific research has taught us more and more about the nature of addiction, treatment has not changed—or has changed very little—to utilize this information.

If addiction is related to brain chemistry, then it seemed to us that to effectively treat addiction we had to find more effective and natural ways to alter the brain's chemistry. David and I began investigating alternative therapies that could be used to restore healthy brain chemistry, thereby aiding addicts in their recovery: nutrition, auricular therapy, acupuncture, and brain-wave biofeedback (neurofeedback) are but a few.

David started taking amino acids—phenylalanine, tyrosine, and glutamine—formulated with certain vitamins. The results were amazing—he experienced significant relief from his symptoms. This made perfect sense because brain chemicals are produced, in large part, from amino acids and vitamins, and addiction and ADHD are related to brain chemistry.

Because of the remarkable changes resulting from taking the amino acid formulation, David began recommending amino acids to addiction clients, most of whom also got positive results. The right combination of amino acids and vitamins delivered to the brain of the addict can restore the balance of neurotransmitters, bringing a sense of well-being and relief from craving.

Eventually, we heard about a clinic in Mexico that was claiming great success over a fifteen-year period using intravenous amino acid therapy to treat addiction. We checked the clinic out and ended up spending many months there observing addicts as they successfully withdrew from a variety of drugs.

Numerous clinics in the United States now offer intravenous amino acid therapy for the treatment of addiction. In our opinion, this is the most effective and remarkable treatment we have encountered. David and I have observed patients going through detoxification from heroin, alcohol, and cocaine with relatively little discomfort. We have seen them emerge from their mental fog, alert and feeling good within days. One of the most remarkable things about amino acid therapy is that many patients report that all craving for the addictive substance disappears. In addition, many indicate that they feel better than they ever felt, suggesting that they had suffered from amino acid and vitamin deficiencies most of their lives.

While searching for more effective treatments, we found that other neurological treatments are currently being used successfully to help people overcome the craving for alcohol or drugs. Hundreds of drug courts throughout the United States have found that auriculotherapy, or ear acupuncture, is more effective than traditional methods alone. Brainwave biofeedback has been found to be effective in changing brainwave patterns so individuals have the power to choose to increase brainwaves that help them relax or concentrate better. Many people find therapeutic massage to be relaxing, soothing, and good for the body.

Through our association with Dr. William Hitt at the clinic in Mexico, Dr. Kenneth Blum, Dr. Charles Gant, Julia Ross, Tamea Sisco, and Dr. James Braly, we have observed or reviewed hundreds of cases in which people have benefited from the use of amino acid therapy, and we strongly believe that it is the best-kept secret related to recovery.

Several years ago, we formed an organization called LifeStream Solutions to support centers that use nutritional and other brain-healing therapies and also to improve and refine intravenous nutritional therapy to integrate nutrients in addition to amino acids. We have recently affiliated with Medaus Compound Pharmacy in Birmingham, Alabama, to provide training for medical professionals and to supply high-quality ingredients for intravenous and oral nutritional therapy.

Somewhere in our journey to find better treatment for the physical symptoms of addiction, we began to lose sight of the importance of the psychological and spiritual needs of the recovering person. The clinic in Mexico had no counseling program, and their emphasis was strictly on changing brain chemistry with intravenous amino acids. The clinic's patients felt so good from the treatment that they believed they were cured forever. Consequently, even though they were advised to get follow-up treatment, most did not. When patients relapsed and returned to the clinic it was usually for further treatment because they did not have the follow-up treatment that would have helped them with other aspects of recovery. We found the same thing with programs that utilized brainwave biofeedback, nutrition, and acupuncture. We realized that treating the brain alone without addressing emotional and spiritual needs was as incomplete as treatment that does not provide healing for the brain.

As more scientific information about the biochemical nature of addiction has become available in recent years, we have seen a growing tendency to treat it with prescription medications.

While medications do address the physiology of addiction, we see this as a step in the wrong direction, because:

• In most cases, medications do not treat the underlying problem.
• Medications often have side effects that become problems themselves or cause the person to stop taking them.
• Medications can become new addictions.
• Perhaps most importantly, certain medications pose a danger if people relapse and drink or use while taking them. The resulting reaction between the drug(s) and the addictive substance could be very harmful, even fatal.

For these reasons, we do not present prescription medication as a recommended strategy for healing the addicted brain. Medications should only be used as a last resort, and then with a great deal of caution.

This book is the culmination of what we have learned so far about complete and lasting addiction recovery. We have searched for explanations as to why addiction recovery is so difficult as well as for treatments that could make recovery easier. This is what we have come to believe as a result of our journey:

• Addiction is primarily a disease of the brain, and the biochemical imbalances associated with it create chronic abstinence symptoms that often lead to relapse.
• For many people, unless proper brain chemistry is restored, staying sober and drug-free means living with emotional pain—anxiety, confusion, and depression. (In fact, 25 percent of recovering alcoholics are reported to eventually commit suicide.)
• Treatment that addresses only the psychological, social, and spiritual issues related to addiction is effective less than

20 percent of the time. Complete treatment for addiction requires combining biochemical treatment for the brain with counseling and education to support lifestyle change.

- Alternative therapies for healing the brain are being used with great success—in particular, intravenous and oral delivery of nutrients, with a recovery rate of 70 to 75 percent—but, unfortunately, few people know about them.
- Healing of the brain must be supported by healing of the spirit.
- Self-care and relapse prevention are essential for comfortable ongoing sobriety.

We are witnessing the birth of what we have been searching for. We are entering a new era of treatment. The work being done now is pioneer work, and, for us, the search for more effective treatment goes on.

Perhaps you suffer from alcoholism or drug addiction and have found no effective treatment. Perhaps you are a parent, husband, wife, son, daughter, or friend of an addict and are living a life of quiet desperation, believing your loved one is hopelessly addicted and can never return to healthful living. Perhaps you are an addiction professional (doing everything you know to do to give life back to people who are addicted) facing, day after day, the reality that the large majority of your addicted clients are relapsing because the treatment you offer has not provided relief from the discomfort that often accompanies abstinence. We hope the message of this book will open the door to new options and new hope for you.

CHAPTER 2

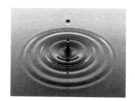

This Is Your Brain on Drugs;
This Is Your Life on Drugs

NO ONE INTENDS TO BECOME ADDICTED. No child says, "I'm going to be an alcoholic when I grow up." No adolescent who experiments with drugs thinks, "I want to become a junkie." No one, when taking the first puff, drink, sniff, or injection, plans on getting addicted to cigarettes, alcohol, marijuana, glue, speed, cocaine, prescription medications, or heroin.

Yet for a great number of people, that first drink or hit leads, deceptively, to physical dependence. It is impossible for anyone who has never been addicted to comprehend the power of addiction. It seems logical and reasonable to stop doing something so harmful to yourself and others, especially those you care about most.

But addicts think about drug use, not with the part of their brain that is reasonable and logical, but with the part that is concerned with survival: the limbic system, the component that tells us to eat, drink, flee, or fight. The limbic system is concerned with keeping us alive. The function of this part of the brain is necessary to keep us alive. It monitors the body's need for survival, and when it senses that our survival is dependent on a certain behavior, it creates a compulsion so strong that it becomes extremely difficult to resist taking that action. Without that compulsion, we might forget to breathe or eat or reproduce.

The limbic system tells addicts that they must have the addictive substance or they will die (and, in some cases, that is true). The limbic system controls the thinking of the addicted person even after the pleasure of drinking or taking drugs has been replaced by severe pain.

Patty, a cocaine addict struggling unsuccessfully to overcome her addiction, describes it this way:

> It seems like I have two brains. There is the brain that tells me that if I use cocaine, I am going to be miserable; it's not fun anymore; it's not worth it; afterward I will feel guilt and remorse and be deeper in debt. The other brain says that I really need this; I have to have it; something worse than death will happen to me if I don't have it; I deserve it; and this time I might get back the old feeling that I need so badly. This argument goes on until the brain in favor of using cocaine convinces the other one that I probably will end up doing it anyway, so I may as well go ahead and do it early so I won't be up all night and unable to work the next day. For some reason, this makes sense to my other brain and I go get some coke.

But how does a person get to the point where the survival part of the brain overrules the reasoning part? And why does it happen to some people who drink alcohol, smoke marijuana, or try cocaine and not happen to others who do the same thing?

James and Richard are brothers we have known since they were young. As teenagers they used drugs together. They used the same drugs in the same quantities. But as they reached college age, James realized that his drug use was interfering with what he wanted out of life. He quit using illegal drugs, though he continued to drink infrequently and always in moderation. By the same age, Richard realized that what he wanted out of life *was* drugs.

James enrolled in college, established a career, had a family, and became a respected, politically active member of his community. Richard also enrolled in college—many times in fact—but he never completed a semester before some drug-related incident interfered and caused him to drop out. He married a couple of times, but when his wives asked him to choose between them and drugs, he chose drugs. He is now in prison, serving an eighteen-month sentence for possession of cocaine.

What was different between these brothers? Why did they take such different paths despite the outward similarities in their early drug use? To answer this, we need to examine what normally happens in the brain and what differs in some people that causes them to be more susceptible to using and becoming addicted to mood-altering substances.

The Reward System of the Brain[1]

We all seek physical and emotional comfort. We want to feel good. It is well established that the action of chemicals in the brain (neurotransmitters) play a significant role in feelings of pleasure and well-being. Manufactured and stored within brain cells (neurons), neurotransmitters carry messages from one neuron to another. When a neuron receives a stimulus (from something we see, hear, feel, smell, think, imagine, or perceive), it sends a chemical message across a synapse (the space between neurons) to receptor sites on the next neuron, which sends the message on to the next. Reaching out like the branches of a tree, each neuron connects with thousands of others, all of which are sending and receiving neurochemical messages from one to another.

Neurotransmitters are chemical messengers that mediate mood, emotion, thought, behavior, motivation, and memories. When neurotransmitters are present in optimal quantities, we have feelings of well-being. Neurotransmitters work together in harmony to create feelings of pleasure to reward us for certain behaviors that help keep us alive and comfortable. A deficiency or excess of any neurotransmitter will give rise to uncomfortable feelings.

Some neurons produce neurotransmitters that *excite* the second neuron while others produce messengers that *inhibit* it. If the neurotransmitter from the first neuron tells the next one to manufacture a substance that makes you feel good, you begin to feel happy and satisfied. But if the message is to stop the production of the feel-good molecule, you begin to feel anxious, irritated, or depressed. You may experience a craving for a mood-altering substance or feel overwhelmed by the stresses and pressures of normal living.

Neurotransmitters are manufactured in the brain's neurons from amino acids. Serotonin, dopamine, norepinephrine, gamma-aminobutyric acid (GABA), taurine, and opioid peptides (endorphins, enkephalins, and dynorphins, also collectively called opioids) are key neurotransmitters significantly involved in the addiction process.

Serotonin

Serotonin improves one's ability to concentrate and boosts feelings of well-being, relaxation, satiation, and security. Low levels can result in depression, sleep problems, poor concentration, confusion, difficulty making decisions, aggressiveness and violence, sugar and carbohydrate cravings, and increased sensitivity to pain.

Dopamine

Dopamine and its derivative norepinephrine stimulate alertness, awareness, wakefulness, and a sense of vitality and energy. They speed up thought processes and improve muscle coordination. Low levels can cause lethargy and weakness, depression, tremors and other movement disorders associated with Parkinson's disease, and many symptoms of attention deficit hyperactivity disorder (ADHD). High levels of dopamine and norepinephrine can result in anxiety, fear, excessive energy, violence, and even schizophrenia and paranoia. When serotonin is low and dopamine is high, you can feel depression and anxiety at the same time.

Opioids

The opioid peptides—endorphins, enkephalins, and dynorphins—are powerful natural pain relievers. They are overproduced in response to pain and physical exertion and block the transmission of pain signals at the receptor site. They also combine with other neurotransmitters to produce feelings of euphoria.

GABA

Popularly referred to as the body's natural tranquilizer, GABA helps to relax the mind, reduce anxiety, and keep stress-related nerve impulses at bay. Normally, the brain produces all the GABA we need, but environmental factors can result in depleted levels of GABA. Too little of this important substance can result in anxiety, irritability, and insomnia. While GABA is sometimes called the natural Valium of the brain, author and clinician Dr. Charles Gant has said that it should be stated the other way around—that Valium should be called the unnatural GABA, because Valium can only temporarily make you feel the way you would if your brain were producing adequate amounts of GABA.

Neurotransmitter Receptors

Once released, neurotransmitters seek out and attach to adjacent neurons that have receptors with a complementary shape. Neurotransmitters fit into these receptors the way a key fits into a lock, and receptors will accept only those neurotransmitters with a corresponding shape. To complicate matters, however, there are three types of receptors for serotonin, five for dopamine, four for noreprinephrine, two for GABA, and five for opioids, plus a number of subtypes. To really understand the addiction process, it is important to understand that the receptors will also accept ingested mood-altering chemicals that mimic natural brain chemicals.

The Reward Cascade

The interactions of neurotransmitters have a powerful effect on our emotions and thinking. As these stimulators and inhibitors act upon one another, a chemical cascade is formed that should create an adequate supply of dopamine in the area of the brain called the nucleus accumbens, often referred to as the reward area of the brain. When this process works as nature intends, this chemical cascade results in feelings of pleasure and well-being.

We choose most of our actions to produce this feeling of reward. We eat because it produces a reward of satiation and pleasure. We eat *certain* foods because they produce a better reward than others (chocolate produces more reward for most people than parsley). We have sex because it creates a powerful release of pleasurable chemicals. We work because the work itself is rewarding for us or because the end result produces a reward. We refrain from certain actions because they do not produce the feeling of reward we are seeking.

When the reward system of the brain is working properly, it creates a sense of well-being, pleasure, and satiation with normal activities. When our needs are met, our brain rewards us. Simple as that. A word of praise for a job well done acts as a stimulus that activates a chemical reaction in the brain that feels good. A hug from a loved one sets off a brain chemical interaction that acts as a reward.

The way we think, feel, and behave results from chemical interactions in the brain and, in turn, produces additional chemical reactions in the brain. When the result of an action is positive, it reinforces that behavior and motivates us to repeat it. We tend to repeat actions that cause us to feel relaxed, happy, satisfied, complete, and fulfilled.

What produces these rewards is different for different people. Chocolate may produce more reward for one person, while potato chips may produce more reward for someone else. Reading a novel may be rewarding for someone, while skiing may be rewarding for another. We all differ in what gives us satisfaction and in the depth of satisfaction we experience. But we are all motivated by chemical actions in the brain that nature uses to keep us alive, motivated, functional, and reproducing.

But what happens if and when this reward system does not work properly?

Reward Deficiency[2]

Some scientists use the term *reward deficiency* to describe a condition in which the reward system of the brain is not working properly and results in lack of reward for normal activities. The body seeks a neurochemical balance, and when there is too much of one neurotransmitter or not enough of another the brain sends out a powerful message to correct the imbalance.

This imbalance of neurotransmitters can result in a reward deficiency that can manifest itself as restlessness, anxiety, emptiness, lack of satisfaction, and vague or specific cravings. These feelings are the brain's message to us to take action to correct the imbalance. People with reward deficiency may feel as if they are constantly in need of something to fill the emptiness, reduce the anxiety, elevate the mood, quiet the restlessness, or satisfy the cravings.

There are numerous causes of reward deficiency in the brain. Many people are born with a genetic impairment that interferes with normal brain chemical balances and interactions. Numerous genes have been identified that are associated with conditions that manifest themselves as symptoms of reward deficiency. Among the genetic conditions associated with reward deficiency are ADHD, Tourette's syndrome, and obsessive-compulsive disorder. And this is a key point: *Many people born with a genetic reward deficiency are also genetically predisposed to addiction.*

Jan's father was an alcoholic. Although she was not aware of it at the time, she realizes now that he also had ADHD. She was diagnosed with ADHD as an adult recovering alcoholic. In remembering her childhood, Jan recalls that she was always restless and anxious, had difficulty concentrating, was easily stressed, and was distracted by noise and competing sounds. She remembers that she never felt comfortable, at ease, or satisfied. She believed there was something seriously wrong with her, but she had no idea what it was. She just knew from an early age that she was different. It wasn't until she discovered alcohol in her early teens and began using it to change her brain chemistry that she began to fit in and feel comfortable and satisfied.

Although the risk of addiction is very high among those who are genetically predisposed, reward deficiency from non-genetic causes can also put a person at high risk for addiction. The normal process of neurotransmission can be altered by environmental conditions as well as genetic.

Prenatal conditions such as alcohol use or drug use by the mother, malnutrition, exposure to toxins, or injury during pregnancy can result in a lifetime of impaired brain chemistry.

Malnutrition over an extended period of time (caused by very-low-calorie dieting, the unavailability of food, food allergy/sensitivity, or a nutritionally inadequate diet) can impair the proper production and interaction of brain chemicals. Neurotransmitters are, after all, produced from amino acids, vitamins, and minerals, most of which are derived from food. When these precursor or building-block nutrients are lacking, the neurotransmitter system breaks down.

Severe or ongoing stress can do long-term damage to the reward system of the brain. This stress may be in the form of a single traumatic event (experiencing an earthquake or witnessing a murder), intermittent or chronic stressful events (child abuse), a series of highly stressful situations (a death followed by a serious injury followed by a job loss), or an ongoing condition of unrelenting stress (living with an alcoholic or drug-addicted person). The importance of extreme stress in relation to altered brain chemistry cannot be overstated. The biochemical reaction to stress is normal and protective. With normal stress, biochemicals return to normal as the stress passes. But when stress is severe or prolonged, chemical levels may never return to normal. And the condition of chronic stress sets the stage for the use of mood-altering substances to lower the stress. This may account for the high number of female addicts who have been sexually abused.

Physical trauma, particularly to the head, can also lead to an imbalance in neurochemicals. Richard, the brother described earlier in this chapter, suffered head trauma at age six, and it was after that that he began showing some of the characteristics that distinguished him from his brother James.

Exposure to environmental toxins such as pesticides and heavy metals can alter brain chemistry.

Heavy or long-term use of mood-altering substances can alter brain chemistry. So people who may not have the genetic predisposition or are not malnourished or traumatized may develop reward deficiency just by their continued use of mood-altering substances. If James had used drugs long enough and heavily enough, he may have altered his brain chemistry as well. This is important when considering the question of who becomes addicted and who doesn't.

For the most part, as we discussed earlier, people who become addicted have a genetic predisposition for it. But that doesn't mean that someone who does not have the genetic predisposition *cannot* become addicted. Whether or not an individual becomes addicted to a substance depends upon the addictiveness of the substance, the frequency and quantity of use, and the susceptibility of the person. Some substances are addictive to almost anyone who uses them. Nicotine is a good example. The majority of people who smoke tobacco for any length of time become addicted and find it very difficult to quit. Many researchers consider nicotine to be more addictive than crack cocaine (unlike alcohol, which is only addictive to about one out of ten people who drink.) It should be noted, however, that some people can smoke without becoming addicted. They do not smoke heavily, and when they decide to quit they throw away their cigarettes and never pick them up again. These people cannot understand why other people cannot do the same. For most people, however, smoking is highly addictive. Some individuals with a certain genetic makeup start smoking at a younger age and find it so difficult to quit that repeated efforts prove futile. They need to be aware that they are not weak-willed. These people need extra help, and some of the measures in this book should be helpful for them.

Whether reward deficiency is caused by genetic or environmental factors, it puts individuals at higher risk for using a substance to relieve the discomfort of the deficiency and also for becoming addicted to that substance. Let's look now at what happens when those with reward deficiency discover a substance that provides what they are missing.

Self-Medicating Reward Deficiency

When the normal process of neurotransmission is disrupted, the resulting state of discomfort can lead to self-medicating with mood-altering substances for relief. Remember that mood-altering substances fit the same receptors as neurotransmitters. So, if there is a deficiency of a natural brain chemical, the newly found substance (whether it's a drug, a food, or behavior) becomes a substitute for the natural chemical, thus, at least temporarily, correcting the deficiency. Suddenly, the anxiety, restlessness, emptiness, and cravings are gone. The reward-deficient person may feel relieved, *normal* for the first time in his or her life. But the substance usually does more than allow the person to feel normal. The brain is flooded with the substance, which produces feelings of intense pleasure and euphoria.[3]

David: In a book I coauthored, *Overload: Attention Deficit Disorder and the Addictive Brain,* I describe my first experience with alcohol when I was about twelve during my uncomfortable life with reward deficiency:

While I was drinking about the third beer, my brain got very excited. It sent me the message that this was the stuff I had been searching for all my life.

"Did you feel what I just felt, old buddy?"

"Yeah, brain, what in the hell was that?"

"That, my dear boy, was the nectar of the gods running through us like a healing stream and taking all our tensions away."

"Yeah, that's what it feels like all right. Kind of like I've been washed clean of all that ails me."

That sense of relief those beers brought was a revelation. I felt free for the first time in my life. . . . In control . . . I knew this was now. I was in this instant, loving this instant of time, never wanting it to go away. The present had always been my enemy, now it was my friend. . . . Alcohol was my ticket to space travel. . . . It was my friend, my lover. . . .

Continued Use and Tolerance

Are reward-deficient individuals more likely than the average person to continue using a mood-altering substance once they have found one that works for them? Of course they are. It is highly unlikely that, having discovered a way to instantly feel better, they will not do it over and over again. That is the reward they have been missing. And just as a hungry person seeks the reward of food, reward-deficient people seek what will satisfy their hunger. And the reward is immediate. They don't have to wait for a payoff. It works, it works now, and it works every time (at least in the beginning). It relieves their discomfort and gives them pleasure. They are no longer reward-deficient. They have discovered a way to feel good.

There are two reasons why people with reward deficiency are likely to become addicted. First is the continued and regular use of the mind-altering substance. The other is that people with genetic reward deficiency are more susceptible to becoming addicted because it seems the same genes that cause reward deficiency also cause something different to occur in their bodies when they use mood-altering substances. They metabolize the substance differently, thereby changing what happens in the brain. The experience for them is not just pleasant but exhilarating. They get a higher high.

For alcoholics, the extreme high is probably due to the interaction of high levels of acetaldehyde.[4] Individuals with a genetic predisposition to become alcoholic do not metabolize alcohol in the same way as other people. They break the alcohol down more slowly. Acetaldehyde, a normal by-product of the breakdown of alcohol in the body, builds up to higher levels in alcoholics than in non-alcoholics. This substance makes its way to the brain and combines with brain chemicals to produce TIQ[5] (see sidebar), a morphine-like substance that is extremely addictive. TIQ not only enables people to feel euphoric but also enables them to function better than normal.

It is very difficult to detect addiction in its early stages because using the substance is more beneficial than harmful for the people who are most susceptible. It provides what their brains normally lack. Just as Ritalin (a mood-altering, amphetamine-like substance) can allow some children with ADHD (a reward-deficiency condition) to function better, other drugs are beneficial for other reward-deficiency conditions. These drugs may make it possible to be more sociable, more at ease, and demonstrate a higher level of social skills. Physical performance may even improve. Contrary to the common belief that consuming increasing quantities of alcohol results in a decreased ability to function, some people may actually perform some tasks better when they're somewhat intoxicated.

Consequently, the earliest warning sign of the onset of addiction (the ability to function well), interferes with early diagnosis and makes it difficult for a developing addict or others to recognize there is a problem. The ability to "hold their liquor" (or nicotine or marijuana or prescription drug) actually conceals the problem and creates the belief among early stage addicts that they are immune to the painful consequences that they see others experience because of drinking or

The Story of Tetrahydroisoquinoline (TIQ)

During World War II, because of the shortage of morphine for pain on the battlefield, a synthetic morphine was developed called tetrahydroisoquinoline (TIQ). It worked well as a pain-killer, but it couldn't be used because it was too addictive. Later, this same substance was found, during autopsies, in the brains of people who had died from alcoholism. It was thought to be morphine. Why would morphine be in the brains of alcoholics? This is not a natural substance produced by the body. But it was not morphine. It was TIQ. Now we know that this substance is created by a metabolic abnormality in alcoholics and people with the genetic predisposition to become alcoholic.

TIQ is created when acetaldehyde (created in excess in alcoholics when they drink) combines with brain chemicals to produce this morphine clone. Most people do not produce TIQ when they drink because the normal metabolic process converts alcohol into acetaldehyde and then breaks it down further as it passes through the body. But with the alcoholic metabolic pathway, the breakdown occurs more slowly and allows a buildup of acetaldehyde, which finds its way to the brain, combines with natural chemicals, and becomes the morphine-like substance TIQ, which produces a high much greater than normal.

For almost anyone, drinking is a pleasant experience. (That is why people drink socially.) But for people with a predisposition to become addicted, the experience is exhilarating and energizing.

drug use. Addiction is a disease that appears to be beneficial in the early stage, allowing the person to experience euphoria without paying any of the penalties.

All the while, however, the brain is changing and adapting to the regular ingestion of the drug. Early on, these changes may seem beneficial. People who are becoming addicted can usually tolerate larger and larger quantities without becoming intoxicated and without experiencing harmful consequences. This is called tolerance.

But over time, continued heavy use, especially by people with a genetic predisposition, leads to addiction. As they are able to consume increasing quantities and their bodies adapt to the presence of these larger quantities, they eventually *must* use even larger quantities to get the same effect, creating more and more changes in the brain.

Jan knew from the first drink that she would continue to use alcohol to feel good. She knew immediately that it took away all the things about her that always made her feel different. At first she could drink with no problems. She could drink more than her friends could without getting drunk. She was able to function better after she had a few drinks than she could sober. She felt more free to express herself. She started writing poetry and thought she had found or released her creative side. She found that as she drank more, she was able to drink even more. She began to find that the amounts she had used before no longer did for her what they used to, and she increased the frequency and quantity of her drinking. She was unaware that biochemical and physical changes were taking place in her brain which were setting her up for problems. She thought she was in no danger of becoming addicted because she could hold her liquor better than anyone she knew. She was not aware that this was an early warning sign of alcoholism. Alcohol was her best friend and, she thought, her friend for life.

Using Addictive Substances to Relieve the Painful Consequences of Using Addictive Substances

When substance use is heavy and continual, the good feelings produced at first are eventually negated by the painful consequences. These consequences can come in many forms. Problems may arise from drinking and driving or other violations of the law. There may be family or job problems. Or there may be physical complications. Whatever the problems are, the user now knows how to make the pain go away. Using the mood-altering substance temporarily takes away pain. So the person, now feeling some painful consequences, uses more and more. The more pain, the more use. The need to use the substance to relieve the pain of using the substance blocks the awareness of what is really causing the pain.

What is happening in the brain at this point is that the mood-altering substance is interfering with the release of neurotransmitters and blocking the receptors. With heavier use, fewer neurotransmitters are being produced and released. And it takes more and more of the substance to fill the receptors and get high.

Let's get back to Jan. To her surprise, she began to have problems because of her drinking. At first, she did not realize that these problems had anything to do with drinking. She began skipping school and thought she was just having a good time. When she was caught and punished at home and suspended from school, she told herself that everyone was just overreacting to her free spirit. She felt misunderstood and angry. What did she do? She comforted herself by drinking more.

Dependence

Addicts are unaware that physiological and biochemical changes are occurring as long as they are able to drink or get their drug. They think they are functioning normally. And they may believe they are drinking or using responsibly or at least attempting to do so. When enough problems occur, addicts may attempt to control their use. But by the time they are aware that their alcohol or other drug use is the problem, they cannot choose to use responsibly. As the brain adapts to higher levels of the substance, the body accepts this as normal and demands that this new state of normal be maintained.

While tolerance is increasing, so is dependence. Want becomes need. The need to use grows. Craving for the substance leads to continued substance use despite the painful consequences. The person cannot function without the substance. The person no longer uses the substance to simply feel good or to relieve the painful consequences caused by the substance. As neurons in the brain adapt to larger and larger quantities, the brain becomes reliant upon the mood-altering substance and shuts down its own production of neurotransmitters. The brain does not need to keep producing neurotransmitters because the receptors are being filled by ingested substances.

When the brain does not get its supply from an outside source, it does not snap into production and start supplying the needed chemicals. It screams out for more of the ingested substance. The addict now uses alcohol or other drugs only to relieve the painful consequences of not using them. This is when the survival part of the brain takes over. It believes it must have the substance to survive. It overpowers the rational part of the brain, and obtaining the substance becomes as strong and vital a need as breathing. Noted journalist Bill Moyers has called this the "hijacked brain." The drug has essentially stolen the addict's ability to think rationally and to choose responsibly.

When Jan got married, her husband objected to her heavy drinking, so she decided she would cut back. But her attempts were short-lived. She would cut back for a few days and then soon find that she was back to her regular amount. As this became more and more of a problem in her marriage, she tried many ways to drink in moderation. She would set rules—then break them. She would promise herself she would only drink during certain times of the day. Or that she would drink only on weekends. Or that she would only drink beer. Or that she would drink only with other people. But she broke every promise she made to her husband and herself. Fearing her husband was going to leave her, Jan promised to quit entirely. And she did. For two days. She was sick and miserable for those two days. She never stopped thinking about drinking. She was obsessed with the idea of having just one. The compulsion to take that one drink was overpowering. Finally, convinced she could have one and stop, she gave in and soon her drinking was out of control again. Not surprisingly, her husband did leave her which provided her a real reason to drink, and alcohol completely took over her life.

The Pleasure Is Gone

What was once the great friend has now become an enemy. The drug no longer produces any pleasure. It creates pain, suffering, and misery. Instead of being able to use more and more, addicts at this point can use less and less before becoming sick, out of control, afraid, and miserable. There is pain when using drugs and pain when not using them. The drug has depleted the brain's supply of natural feel-good chemicals and the drug is no longer a satisfactory substitute. Addicts continue to use alcohol or other drugs, not for any pleasure, but only because the survival part of the brain has taken over and believes it must have the substance or die. Attempts to stop are usually short-lived and futile. Severe anxiety results when an unexpected situation interferes with the substance use or the source of supply.

At this point, many of the addict's family, friends, and associates believe the person is behaving irresponsibly, unaware that the person is not choosing the behavior—that it is being dictated by the survival part of the brain. It takes less and less of the substance before the person loses control and experiences symptoms of intoxication. The person may go immediately from the pain of needing the drug to the pain of using the drug. The magic is gone. The pleasure is gone. There is nothing but pain. Pain while not using the substance. Pain while using it.

Jan doesn't remember when the pleasure stopped and drinking brought her only pain. At first she thought she was so miserable because her husband had left her. Gradually she became aware that drinking was giving her no comfort. She was getting drunk more and more often. She could drink less and less before getting sick. Where had the magic gone? She was convinced she could find it again if she could just find the secret door. She tried to work at several jobs but was too sick most of the time to go to work. She was lonely and started going out with friends with whom she previously drank, those people who used to comment about her ability to hold her liquor. But now she was passing out and they were driving her home. They didn't like being with her anymore. Every day she would promise herself that tomorrow she would stop. But tomorrow she only remade the promise.

Eventually Jan was able to get sober with the help of Alcoholics Anonymous. But it was the hardest thing she ever did, and now she lives one day at a time, recognizing that she can never learn to drink in moderation. Jan still grieves the loss of her best friend, alcohol. She yearns for the comfort it gave her and is looking for something else that might give her some of the pleasure she found in drinking.

Abstinence

There are times when addicted people may have a moment of sanity and realize that if they keep using they will die. Thus, they may ask for help. They may enter a treatment center. If it is a treatment center without medical detoxification, the pain of abstinence is so severe that addicts frequently leave before they have made it all the way through the detoxification process. If they receive medical detoxification, many stick it out even though they are uncomfortable. But what happens now to the poor brain, totally depleted of natural brain chemicals and unable to produce an adequate supply? Usually nothing. It stays that way. Perhaps for months, perhaps for years. It is reward-deficient. Even more so than before drinking or drug use began.

What was discomfort prior to substance use now is even more intense. And the brain continues to crave the substance upon which it has come to depend. After struggling through months of pain, misery, and craving, many addicts give up in despair, and believing there is no way out, go back to what they know will at least relieve the craving, if not the pain.

Over a period of thirteen years, Mark, a heroin addict we met while he was getting intravenous nutrient therapy, attempted recovery many (he thinks as many as fifty) times. Sometimes he left before he got through detox and went right back to using heroin. Sometimes he made it through a thirty-day treatment program and stayed clean for a while. Always during his periods of sobriety, he went to twelve-step meetings. But he was totally depleted of energy. He says he was so lethargic that sometimes he couldn't get out of bed. He did not have the energy to work at his job in construction. Sometimes he thought he might have some kind of illness but nothing was ever diagnosed. Finally, believing he would never be able to function normally again, he would give up and go back to heroin. No matter how hard he tried, he was never able to maintain more than thirty days of sobriety. That is, until he received intravenous nutrient treatment that changed his brain chemistry and provided relief from the pain of abstinence and gave him the energy he needed to function normally.

Now, many people will tell you that Mark was just not motivated to get sober—that if he *really* wanted to, he could do it. But why would he go to treatment over and over again, usually voluntarily, unless he really wanted to free himself from his addiction? Remember that he had been in treatment as many as fifty times. Why would you attempt something for the fiftieth time—you had already failed forty-nine previous times—if you didn't really want it? Some people might say that Mark just hadn't hurt enough yet. No, it was not the lack of pain that kept him locked into his addiction. *It was too much pain.* It was not until his brain was healed and he was relieved of his pain that he was able to live a normal life. Some people will tell you that Mark just did not have any self-discipline. How many of us have the self-discipline to endure ongoing, unrelenting pain without relief—and no relief in sight—without looking for some source of pain relief?

Let us be clear here that many addicted people do make it and find ways to maintain sobriety. Many find a better life through practicing the program of a twelve-step group. Thousands of recovering people are living proof that sobriety and recovery from addiction are possible. Through their experience of addiction and recovery they find meaning and purpose and are able to live in serenity and peace. *We are concerned for those who do not find this path.* While some do find relief from their addictions, the majority of those who are addicted do not. Their craving brains interfere with their ability to follow the road that has led to recovery for others.

So, for someone experiencing the discomfort and/or pleasure deficit of imbalanced neurochemistry, mood-altering chemicals do, for a period of time, work to bring relief and feelings of pleasure and well-being. But eventually the good feelings of self-medication are replaced by the pain of addiction. What starts out as a rewarding experience—and perhaps an improvement in the ability to function—becomes a dependence on the substance in order to function. This happens as the drug further impairs the reward system of the brain and further impairs neurological functioning. The impairment may be so severe that the person is physically, emotionally, and mentally unable to function without the drug. The need to use the drug overpowers normal reasoning and previous life values.

When the addict attempts to abstain, craving for the substance to relieve the pain of impaired neurochemistry during withdrawal leads the person back to use of the substance over and over again. Therefore, relapse is common and may lead to feelings of hopelessness and the belief that sobriety is impossible. Many addicts give up and finally experience physical, economic, and social deterioration or—too frequently—death.

Attempting recovery from addiction, then, without addressing the neurological pain and craving that accompany it, is much like attempting recovery from diabetes without addressing the health of the pancreas. Most treatment is helpful in that it helps addicts cope with the craving and pain of abstinence, but does not take it away.

With our current scientific information, more options are becoming available to rebalance brain chemistry and restore normal neurotransmission, thus relieving the craving and discomfort of abstinence. This frees the addict to focus on other necessary tasks of recovery: rebuilding a damaged and impaired life and developing a new lifestyle that will support the maintenance of healthy brain chemistry.

Behavioral Addictions

There are two types of triggers for addiction: mood-altering substances and mood-altering activities or behaviors. The process of addiction as we have described it can result from excessive ingestion of substances such as alcohol, cocaine, heroin, marijuana, nicotine, sugar, or any number of prescription drugs. The same process can occur as a result of excessive behaviors or activities. Behaviors that can become excessive and compulsive, and therefore addictions, include gambling or risk-taking, working or achieving, excessive sexual activity, excessive spending or compulsive spending, and certain eating behaviors. They can also include a relationship that becomes excessive or compulsive, playing computer games or racing cars or golfing or running. It is not so much what you do as how you do it. You may wonder how an activity can change brain chemistry if nothing is ingested to bind to the receptor sites as a mood-altering substance does. The explanation lies in a better understanding of the relationship between body and mind.

All our thoughts, feelings, and actions affect brain chemistry; and brain chemistry affects our thoughts, feelings, and actions. You have no doubt heard about the power of positive thinking. There is also power in negative thinking. Happy thoughts as well as angry, sad, or worry thoughts cause a release of chemicals in the body. Were you ever in physical or emotional pain and then smiled because of something cute your child or pet did and then realized that your pain was diminished? Were you ever feeling great and then happened to think about some disturbing situation that caused you to feel tired or perhaps develop a headache? These are examples of the power of our thoughts and feelings.

Even more powerful than thoughts and feelings are our actions. How did you feel? Research shows that a full body laugh changes your brain chemistry for up to forty-five minutes. We refer to these as endogenous opioids because the release is not triggered by something you consume; it comes from within.

There are activities that change our biochemistry so much that we want to do them over and over. Some people get a biochemical response from shoplifting or inappropriate sex that is equal to or greater than a heroin injection. Nature has given us natural opioids in the brain to mediate pain. These neurotransmitters work to relieve physical as well as emotional pain. People born with the inability to feel good will look for ways to stimulate the release of these chemicals—and that often includes video games, shoplifting, gambling, inappropriate sex and so on.

The opioids that are released from risk-taking or sex are metabolized through the same dopamine pathway as cocaine or heroin or alcohol. And if the person has a reward deficit that predisposes to addiction, the activity that works will be repeated as often as necessary to get the desired reward. For the person predisposed to addiction the chosen activity will rapidly proceed from self-medication to addiction.

Work addiction is fairly common in our society because over-working is applauded and rewarded. And the painful consequences of overworking may not be as apparent or recognized as activities that do not have the same kind of social payoff. But work addiction is not the same as the compulsion to achieve. Some people get their biochemical payoff from the act of working while other people get it from the resulting accomplishments.

Risk-taking and gambling addiction are pretty much the same addiction. That is one of the reasons that this is such a difficult behavior to control; it just changes forms. For some people gambling addiction takes the form of shoplifting or other unlawful behaviors that carry a risk of getting caught. The euphoria of shoplifting does not lie in the item taken but in the mood-altering event of taking it. If the item were free the act of taking it simply would not provide the same payoff.

A Story of Gambling and Risk-taking Addiction

Curt developed an addiction to casino gambling. His family and friends were quite astonished by this behavior because even gambling on cards was not customary for him. A friend talked him into going to the casino the first time where he discovered a game that was a combination of skill and luck, and the challenge of it hooked him immediately. He won and it was exhilarating. He went back the next night—and the next. It was not long before he found himself thinking about and anticipating going again.

Before long, Curt was leaving work during the day and neglecting his business. He was on a winning streak, and his euphoria was beyond anything he had ever experienced with any kind of substance. When he began losing, he was sure that the next time he would make it back. It was not until his wife threatened to leave him that he went to Gamblers Anonymous and with a great struggle gave up the casino. The craving was intense. He was soon satisfying this craving with cars. He started buying cars—Porches, Lamborghinis, and Aston Martins—and driving them 120 miles an hour. In the state where he lived this is a felony and he found himself in trouble with the law. That is when he realized that he had not stopped gambling; it had just taken another form.

Sex addiction. Like other behaviors that can become an addiction, sexual activity is a normal and healthy activity. But when it becomes compulsive and obsessive, it becomes harmful. When people risk other things of value to satisfy the need for out-of-bounds sexual activity, then that activity has become an addiction and requires help.

Food addiction is a combination of mood-altering substances and mood-altering behaviors. Food can contain any number of mood-altering substances, but failure to eat (anorexia) and purging (bulimia) are mood-altering activities. Karen Carpenter, the singer from the Carpenters who died as a result of anorexia and bulimia, once said that she got high from the feeling of an empty stomach. Even excessive dieting that does not reach the level of anorexia can be mood-altering and addictive.

Prescription Medications?

Prescription drugs are not the answer to addiction because, in most cases, they do not treat the underlying problem. They often have side effects that become problems themselves or cause the person to stop taking them. A common problem is that many of the drugs used to treat addiction are addictive. There is no point in trading one addiction for another. And prescription drugs can pose a danger if people have a relapse of their primary addiction and have the medication in their system. Combining mood-altering substances can create a life-threatening synergistic effect in the body. And there way be unexpected reactions to some substances. For example, there are medications that are or will be prescribed for addiction that block the effects of certain addictive substances by blocking the pleasure centers of the brain. But these substances may also block the ability to get pleasure in other ways and lead to depression or thoughts of suicide. Before any prescription drugs are used all other natural methods should be tried. Every day you read of deaths because of prescription drugs. We know of no deaths due to any of the methods that we recommend.

A Story of Addiction

Fred began drinking mouthwash when he was four or five years old. He was a restless, impulsive child. Drinking mouthwash made him feel good. When he was ten he found a bag of marijuana his father had taken from an older brother. He replaced the marijuana in the bag with parsley and smoked the marijuana. It made him feel great. From that day on he smoked marijuana daily. He knew from early childhood that mood-altering substances would be an important part of his life. But it never occurred to him that there might come a time when drugs might become an enemy rather than a friend.

Fred stayed high on marijuana or alcohol most of the time throughout his childhood. Even so, he maintained good grades with little effort. His family and teachers had no idea he was hiding such a habit. In ninth grade he began using speed (amphetamine) and crack cocaine. He was still able to function all right. He was part of a very wealthy family, so getting money for the drugs was never a problem.

Fred had only good experiences with drugs until he started using a needle. He says that nothing was ever the same again. The rush from injected drugs was the most important thing in his life. By that time he was around twenty. Soon he was speedballing (using cocaine and heroin together). Daily use caused him no problems for about nine months. Then his friend very rapidly became his enemy. There was no longer pleasure from the drugs. He was sick and miserable.

Fred knew he needed to get off the heroin and cocaine, so he decided to try treatment. He stopped using heroin and cocaine (detoxed with Librium). He continued to smoke marijuana during treatment and never intended to give up marijuana and alcohol. After eighteen days he was feeling fine and decided he didn't need any more treatment and abruptly left the treatment center. Four months later he was again injecting 3.5 grams of cocaine and 3 grams of heroin daily.

At this point Fred knew he was in deep trouble and thought there was no way out. A large inheritance made it easy to keep doing what he was doing. He came to the conclusion that he was one of those people who was on earth to live fast and die young. He deteriorated rapidly. He was part of what he calls a ruthless drug scene. He was sharing needles, shooting up crack. It didn't take long to go through his inheritance. So he tried working for his brother for awhile. But it was physical labor and he was in bad physical condition. He was 6'2" yet weighed only 155 pounds. He was weak and sweating within a half-hour of beginning work. But he had to wear long sleeves to cover the needle marks. He was always late and took bathroom breaks every twenty minutes. So much for trying to work.

By the time Fred had been injecting drugs seven years he says he found it quite ironic that his mother was a millionaire and he had turned into a bum. "I could have had anything I wanted, but I didn't want anything but drugs." He was living in his truck, shooting up while driving. He was getting no pleasure from the drugs; he was just trying to stay alive and truly believed he would die without them. At the same time he knew he was going to die if he kept on the road he was on. Six of his friends had died within the previous year. He thought there was no way out. No hope. Just waiting to die.

Periodically Fred would see his mother to get money. One day she was crying and told him she knew what he was doing. He told her he didn't know any other way to live. She told him of a treatment she had heard about that might work for him. She begged him to try. He agreed to go after the holidays. Four hours later he was sitting in jail. He had been stopped by the police with needles and spoons all over his truck. Though drugs were hidden in his socks, they weren't found so he was charged with nineteen misdemeanors but no felonies. His mother posted bond and took him directly to treatment where, very near death, he received intravenous nutrient therapy.

After a few uncomfortable days Fred began to notice some remarkable changes. He had clarity of thought he had never experienced in his life. The intense craving for drugs disappeared. After several months he says he can think about drugs without craving them. He feels no need for substitute drugs. Fred began attending twelve-step meetings and he has started college. He enjoys surfing and playing basketball and just being physically active. Fred feels that he has a real life, something he thought he could never have. He says he has goals — which he never had before. At age twenty-seven, he feels he has just been born.

CHAPTER 3

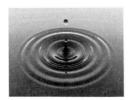

The Pain of Ineffective
Treatment and Relapse

ADDICTION TO ALCOHOL AND OTHER DRUGS takes its toll on
the lives of those who are addicted and their families and on
society as a whole. It kills by overdose, by accidents, by suicides,
by homicides, by destroying the mind and body, and by causing other diseases that disable and kill. It tears apart families,
fills our prisons, steals our children, and drains our economy.
Consider the following:[1]

- Our nation's drug problem costs $70 billion per year. This
  figure includes legal, medical, and treatment costs; the cost
  of lost productivity on the job; the cost of drug-related
  crime; and the cost of social programs that address poverty,
  child and spouse abuse, and other social issues that result
  directly and indirectly from addiction.
- More than one-half of all people brought into the criminal
  justice system suffer from some form of addiction.

- 3.5 million Americans are chronic drug users.
- 1 million Americans are in addiction treatment.
- There are 1 million drug arrests per year.
- 60 percent of all federal prisoners are drug offenders.
- 31 percent of all felony convictions in 1994 were for drug offenses.
- 75 percent of all prison growth since 1980 is due to drug offenders.
- Alcohol and other drugs are associated with
    - –36 percent of child abuse
    - –52 percent of rapes
    - –62 percent of assaults
    - –20 to 35 percent of suicides
    - –50 percent of spousal abuse
    - –50 percent of traffic fatalities
    - –40 percent of murders
    - –88 percent of manslaughter charges
    - –69 percent of drownings.
- Drug use is the overall leading cause of death in the United States.

We know you are thinking that we are wrong about the above statement because drug and alcohol use is listed by the government behind cancer and heart disease as a leading cause of death. But cancer death rates *include* lung cancer deaths due to nicotine addiction and pancreatic and liver cancer deaths due to alcoholism. Heart disease death rates include deaths from heart problems due to heroin and cocaine addiction. Diabetes death rates include deaths from complications of alcoholism. Adding homicides, suicides, and accidents attributable to alcohol and drug use, it can easily be seen that alcohol and other drug use is *the* leading cause of death in the nation.

Yet while progress has been made in the treatment of cancer, heart disease, and diabetes, little has been done to improve the dismal rates of recovery from addiction, whether addiction to alcohol, nicotine, illegal drugs, or prescription drugs. Little or no progress has been made in the effectiveness of treatment for alcoholism and other drug addictions in the last forty years. Although there are not consistent and accurate methods of attaining addiction recovery and relapse rates, statistics indicate that the recovery rate has not changed much in the last thirty years and claims less than a 20 percent success rate. However, there is no health problem more serious or more widespread.

Is Lack of Treatment the Problem?

Lack of available treatment is often blamed for the cost of addiction to individuals and to society. And it is true—there is a shortage of treatment. From treatment professionals, from those pushing for treatment rather than incarceration, and from those wanting more tax dollars we often hear the phrase "treatment works." We have even heard this from a president of the United States. *But if available treatment is effective for only a small percentage of the people who get it, then we need more than additional treatment; we need better, more effective treatment.* In the treatment of addiction, we are doing the same thing over and over, trying for a different result rather than looking for better answers. Albert Einstein said that the definition of insanity is doing the same thing over and over again and expecting different results. So if you always do what you always did, you'll always get what you always got.

Although there is a scarcity of treatment, this is not the major reason for the severe problems related to addiction in the United States. *Relapse* is the major reason for the high rate of social, medical, and personal problems associated with addiction. Most people who enter conventional treatment centers will relapse, usually more than once, often repeatedly. Effective treatment would reduce relapse rates and improve the quality of sobriety, as well as reduce the destruction that results from addiction.

There is little understanding of addiction or how to treat it by those who most often encounter it: health professionals, human service workers, and those in the criminal justice system. Courses in addiction are seldom taught in medical schools, nursing schools, or schools of theology. Nor are they taught in psychology, social work, or criminal justice programs in colleges and universities. Addiction professionals often don't have a college degree, and they draw largely from their own experience or from what has been done in the past (with a recovery rate of less than 20 percent).

While acknowledging that addiction is truly a physical disease—with profound psychological and social consequences—addiction professionals have primarily addressed the *consequences,* directing little treatment toward the physical disease itself or its underlying causes. Most addiction professionals have recognized that it is a disease but many don't really understand *how* it is a disease or how it comes about; therefore, they don't know how to treat the condition directly. Consequently, the main goal of conventional treatment has been to teach people how to accept and cope with their symptoms.

On the other hand, there are a few treatment centers that do focus on physical recovery, most of which, unfortunately, do not emphasize the other aspects of wellness. Addiction is a physical condition with psychological, behavioral, social, and spiritual consequences. The first step is to treat the unhealthy neurochemistry and physiology of the brain, but treatment that ends there is incomplete. The addict is left with life deficits that cannot be overcome by fixing the brain alone. Even more of a problem is the growing tendency by health professionals to treat addiction with prescription (often mood-altering) medications. Even when used along with counseling and support groups, this practice doe not improve recovery rates.

Symptoms that Interfere with the Ability to Stay Sober

Perhaps what is least understood about the nature of addiction is that there are painful symptoms that occur during abstinence that interfere with the ability to stay sober: craving, stress sensitivity, anxiety, dysphoria, depression, mental confusion, inability to concentrate, increased pain sensitivity, sleep disturbances, and hypersensitivity to the environment.[2]

Most people are unaware that the pain of staying sober can be, and frequently is, so severe that it interferes with the ability to function even when the desire for and commitment to recovery is strong. This chronic discomfort is what leads to relapse.

Most addiction treatment is beneficial in the limited sense that it teaches coping skills for living with the craving and the pain of abstinence. But it does not take them away. While this approach helps many people stay sober, for the majority—those with severe chronic abstinence symptoms—it is not enough. Some hang on; some find substitute addictions; most relapse. Two out of three addicts who enter treatment will relapse, usually within the first three to four months. Some who struggle unsuccessfully may go through treatment twenty—even fifty—times. (Unfortunately, after a couple of failures, they may be refused admittance to some treatment centers.) Their desire to maintain sobriety is strong, so strong that they keep trying over and over again, even after repeated unsuccessful attempts.

While scientific research has opened doors to new understanding of the nature of addiction and its effect on the brain, medical and addiction professionals have applied little of this information to actually helping people get well from this devastating disease. There is a gap between what is known about addiction and what is done about it.

The Contribution of Alcoholics Anonymous

Before Alcoholics Anonymous (AA) was started in the 1930s, alcoholism was considered a hopeless condition. Rarely did anyone recover. Bill Wilson certainly seemed hopeless. He had tried all the cures available, but sobriety always eluded him. After an experience he called a spiritual awakening and involvement in the Oxford Group where he became acquainted with and began to practice some principles for spiritual living, he was able to get a foothold on sobriety. But when he was sent to Akron, Ohio, on an extended business trip, he found himself craving alcohol and sorely tempted to take a drink. Instead, he asked around to find another alcoholic and was directed to a physician, Dr. Bob, who was receptive to the message of the Oxford Group. By sharing his story, Bill was able to avoid a return to drinking, and the fellowship of Bill and Bob was the beginning of the fellowship of Alcoholics Anonymous (AA).

In the years since, AA had spread all over the world and has become the means of recovery for thousands and thousands of alcoholics. The program has been applied to other addictions in the form of Narcotics Anonymous, Overeaters Anonymous, Smokers Anonymous, Sexual Addicts Anonymous, Gamblers Anonymous, and many more.

What does AA offer that has enabled so many people to become sober when they otherwise couldn't? For some it is simply the fellowship, having others available that have walked the same path and are willing and available to help. For some, it's working the twelve steps, which include acceptance of powerlessness over alcohol, willingness to accept help from a higher power, acknowledge and admitting character defects, making amends for wrongdoings, taking regular moral inventory, promptly admitting wrongs, maintaining contact with a higher power through prayer and meditation, and carrying the message of AA to others. For many it is the combination of this change of life focus and the support of other recovering people that provides the strength to put one foot in front of the other until the road becomes smoother.[3] To contact Alcoholics Anonymous, check your local phonebook.

The 12 Steps of Alcoholics Anonymous

1. We admitted we were powerless over alcohol, that our lives had become unmanageable.
2. Came to believe that a power greater than ourselves could restore us to sanity.
3. Made a decision to turn our will and our lives over to the care of God as we understood Him.
4. Made a searching and fearless moral inventory of ourselves.
5. Admitted to God, to ourselves, and to another human being the exact nature of our wrongs.
6. Were entirely ready to have God remove all these defects of character.
7. Humbly asked Him to remove our shortcomings.
8. Made a list of all persons we had harmed and became willing to make amends to them all.
9. Made direct amends to such people wherever possible, except when to do so would injure them or others.
10. Continued to take personal inventory and when we were wrong promptly admitted it.
11. Sought through prayer and meditation to improve our conscious contact with God, as we understood Him, praying only for knowledge of His will for us and the power to carry that out.
12. Having had a spiritual awakening as the result of these steps, we tried to carry this message to alcoholics, and to practice these principles in all our affairs.

The Disease Model of Addiction[4]

From its earliest days, Alcoholics Anonymous has embraced the concept that some people are able to drink alcohol without becoming addicted while others are not; and those unable to control what happens when they drink must remain abstinent. This is the underlying concept that is referred to as the disease model of addiction and is the basis of traditional treatment.

There are several hallmarks of the disease model of alcoholism. The first, as we have just stated, is that the distinction between social drinking and alcoholism lies in the person, not in the substance. Originally it was not known what this was within individuals that set them apart, but it has always been assumed that it was biological rather than psychological. It has sometimes been called an allergy, and while it is not, it is comparable. Most people can eat and enjoy peanuts with no problem. A few people (about one in 250) experience a dangerous reaction to peanuts (hives, difficulty breathing, severe swelling, loss of consciousness) that can even be life threatening. The difference lies in the biological makeup of the people eating the peanuts.

Another basic tenet of the disease model is that once a person has become an alcoholic that person can never learn to drink in moderation; therefore total abstinence is necessary. The preponderance of the evidence shows this to be true.

Yet, while recognizing addiction as a physiological, biochemical abnormality rather than a psychological problem, because of a lack of methods to treat the disease *directly*, the disease model of treatment has consisted mainly of strategies for changing beliefs, attitudes, thinking, behavior, and spiritual principles. This enables people to cope with the disease, but does not change physiology or biochemistry. These principles have proved effective for thousands of people and enabled many to stay sober who otherwise could not. Without these contributions, attitudes toward addiction and treatment might have remained in the dark ages and in the same category as blood-letting. But these are principles for living, not treatment for a disease, and they do not address the underlying neurochemical condition that accompanies addiction. They are methods of coping with the condition, not treating it.

This psychological, social, and spiritual approach to inter-rupting active addiction works for less than 20 percent of those who receive it. And, understandably, those 20 percent become the spokespersons for this approach to recovery. The belief that it is effective for anyone who truly wants to recover and who works the program has become the underpinning for addiction treatment as most people know it. There is an abundance of treat-ment programs built upon this foundation. The scarcity lies in the availability of treatment for the 80 percent who do not recover and are then blamed for their own failure. These relapsers believe what they have been told by the 20 percent—that the failure lies in them, not in the treatment. *We speak for this silent majority.*

For the 80 percent who relapse, working the conventional program has not enabled them to maintain sobriety. And many, while abstinent, have lived lives of quiet agony, never able to find comfort without the drug that once had provided it. For them, pain accompanies the choice to stop using the sub-stance—during the period of acute withdrawal symptoms and for months and years—even decades—into sobriety.

A word from David: When I first made a sincere commitment to quit drinking, I tried a variety of things to help me. I found that I could not do it with willpower, no matter how I tried. I went through an outpatient program at the VA hospital where I got Mellaril (a powerful mood-altering prescription medication) and ping-pong therapy. Not very successful. Not successful at all. I finally agreed to go to an Alcoholics Anonymous meeting. Everyone there was older than I was, and I didn't identify with their war stories. So I didn't go back—until I was in danger of losing my family and realized nothing else was working. I went back with a different attitude. And after a few relapses was able to stay sober. I remember how proud I was when I was recognized at AA for one year of sobriety. What a milestone. But it was a tough year. Even with all the help I had from my AA family I struggled with stress sensitivity, emotional overreaction, cravings, and—long before I had a name for it or a way to describe it—stimulus augmentation.

With Merlene's help I found many ways of coping one day at a time. Nutrition, exercise, plenty of sleep, escape time, and participation in a church community all helped me hang on and work the program of AA. It was years later, when I started taking amino acid supplements, that I found real relief from chronic abstinence symptoms. I am thankful for the freedom that amino acid therapy brought into my life. I will be forever grateful to AA because without it I would never have made it to that point. But I understand the pain that leads people back to drinking or using drugs when AA is not enough to heal the broken brain.

Chronic Abstinence Symptoms of Addiction

Painful symptoms of addiction can occur when someone is using, symptoms that motivate the person to give up addictive use. When the pain becomes severe enough, addicted people usually choose recovery. Recovery requires abstinence, but abstinence triggers new symptoms—or the return of old symptoms that preceded the addiction. Some symptoms pass within a few days, but some emerge and grow more severe as acute withdrawal symptoms subside. Long-term and excessive use of addictive substances causes nutrient depletion and tissue and cellular damage that create reward deficiency or intensify the problems of reward deficiency that existed before addictive use began. So when addictive use stops, the symptoms that led to self-medicating with a mood-altering substance return with greater intensity.

The pain of abstinence usually takes the form of severe anxiety or depression, trouble concentrating and remembering, inability to manage stress, sleep problems, lack of energy, overwhelming cravings, and heightened sensitivity to sights, sounds, touch, and pain.

Stimulus Augmentation

Stimulus augmentation is one term that's used to describe heightened sensitivity to external and internal stimuli. Sometimes it is referred to as hyper-augmentation, hypersensitivity, or simply augmentation. People with this condition are unable to filter out background noises and happenings and feel bombarded by all that is going on around them. They augment or magnify sounds, sights, touch, pain, perceptions, and stress. They feel constantly overwhelmed by everything going on around them and everything going on inside of them. What would usually be considered mild stress is major stress. Sounds that others do not notice are major distractions. Pain is more intense. Being touched can sometimes feel like being mauled. People with this condition feel overwhelmed by a world that comes at them full force.

In most cases this symptom is genetic. Alcoholics, children of alcoholics, and those with ADHD have all been found to magnify perceptual input and this has been associated with craving for alcohol. Stimulus augmentation exists prior to addiction and probably contributes to the risk that someone will use mood-altering substances at an early age.

Inability to Concentrate

An inability to concentrate is a natural result of stimulus augmentation. When the buzzing of a fly demands as much attention as the person talking to you, it is difficult to stay focused on what that person is saying. It is not rudeness; it is not intentional. It is just very difficult to maintain a focus when

Stimulus Augmentation and Alcohol

One researcher who has contributed much to our understanding of stimulus augmentation is Ralph Tarter, director of the Center for Education and Drug Abuse Research (CEDAR). He and his colleagues discovered that alcoholics and children of alcoholics are frequently augmenters (people with stimulus augmentation). But when given alcohol they become what he calls reducers; they no longer magnify input but minimize it. The effect is immediate. The relief is profound. Is it to be expected that when augmenters discover that alcohol (or cocaine, or whatever the drug) reduces the ongoing, unrelenting noise, stress, pain, and confusion of an overwhelming world, they will use that substance again for relief? Of course! Is it reasonable to expect that they will use it again and again? Sure! If a person finds mood enhancement through the use of addicting drugs, the "synthetic" but nevertheless reinforcing reward will motivate that person to more mood-altering drug use. The self-medicating process that begins with a simple need to feel better can easily lead to addiction and complicate an already vexing problem. But what happens when that person recognizes the need to give up the mood-enhancing substance? The pre-existing augmentation returns along with more intense cravings and the augmented brain begs for relief.

everything around you is calling to you at the same time with the same urgency. It can be frustrating and embarrassing to realize that someone is talking to you and you have no idea what they just said.

Memory Problems

Memory problems result from the inability to concentrate. If you didn't hear it or were distracted when it occurred, you won't remember it, or the memory will be sketchy. You can't recall what was never really recorded in your brain in the first place.

Anxiety

Anxiety is common during recovery. Of course, a certain amount of psychological stress is expected because of so much change going on. Change is stressful, and it is normal to have some fear connected with all the changes necessary to make recovery possible. But stress is exacerbated to the point of anxiety by stimulus augmentation, the inability to concentrate, and memory problems.

Dysphoria

Dysphoria is a general feeling of discomfort or unpleasantness. It is the absence of pleasure from doing things that would normally be pleasurable. It can range from mild to severe and is characterized by listlessness and lack of motivation and, sometimes, hopelessness. Ongoing dysphoria takes the color out of life and puts sobriety in jeopardy. Sometimes the dysphoria comes and goes and takes the form of mood swings. Sometimes you feel good and then soon feel very down. The tendency for you and the people around you is to believe when you are feeling good that you are always going to feel good; it is then quite disheartening when you are again overcome by dysphoria.

Drug Hunger (Craving)

Intense craving, or what some refer to as drug hunger, is a powerful compulsion to alter one's mood with a psychoactive drug. Stimulus augmentation has been linked to a strong craving for alcohol, and alcohol normalizes it. The sober person experiencing cravings knows what will bring relief. Most addicts and alcoholics, while actively drinking or using as well as when abstinent, have notoriously poor eating habits and may not realize the profound effect that these eating habits have upon their neurochemistry. Poor nutrition can lead to neurochemical imbalances and erratic blood sugar levels that can be triggers for drug hunger. Feeling incomplete or inadequate or unfulfilled is common with abstinence. There is a feeling of emptiness and a yearning for something—anything—to fill up the emptiness. The emptiness begs for self-medication.

To evaluate the severity of your abstinence symptoms, see the Chronic Abstinence Symptom Severity Scale in Appendix B.

The Stress of Sobriety

Stress intensifies all the symptoms of abstinence. When you make a commitment to sobriety, everything in your life changes, and change is always stressful. In addition, dealing daily with stimulus augmentation, the inability to concentrate, memory problems, mood swings, and cravings creates additional stress.

In handling stress the brain uses large quantities of neurochemicals. Persistent, ongoing stress not only raises the level of stress hormones, but depletes the brain of key neurochemicals, especially the opioids. So during recovery when you are expected to be getting better, the stress of abstinence may actually make you feel worse. People tell you to just hang on and things will get better, but they don't. The daily stress of maintaining abstinence (plus the high levels of stress hormones) may be further depleting your neurotransmitter stores. During times of stress the body releases chemicals to help us keep functioning, but the constant excess of these chemicals can cause irritability, sleeplessness, depression, anxiety, and eventually physical illnesses (high blood pressure, heart disease, and gastrointestinal problems, to mention a few), all of which become new stressors.

Sobriety: Is It Really This Difficult?

I've been sober for a few months, but my brain just feels numb—I don't know how to think or what to think or even if I want to think.

I haven't had a drink in seven weeks, but I feel like I'm going nuts. When my kids yell at each other, I want to curl up into a ball and die. Bright lights, loud noises, intense emotions—I can't be around them. I feel like they are frying my brain.

I'm sober, but my memory is shot, and I'm afraid I have permanent brain damage or maybe even Alzheimer's.

I can't figure it out. I've got eight months of sobriety under my belt, but the anxiety and the fear just don't quit. Once or twice a week I wake up in a sweat, dreaming about the time I ran over my son's bicycle when I was drunk and imagining that I killed him.

Some days I feel great, happy, solidly sober, but then the next day I feel just plain awful. My mood swings are like flash floods—there's never any warning.

I cry all the time. I'm always overreacting to everything—a pile of dirty clothes in the hallway is enough to make me want to scream.

I'm telling you—alcoholism was hell. But what is this, purgatory?

From *Beyond the Influence* [6]

"Constitutionally Incapable of Rigorous Honesty"

While it offers hope, the book *Alcoholics Anonymous* (commonly referred to as "The Big Book"[5]) states that there are people that the program doesn't help. The book says this is not their fault because they are constitutionally incapable of being rigorously honest. Well, why would some be *constitutionally* incapable of being rigorously honest, and why would that interfere with a sincere effort to maintain sobriety?

The answer lies in what we call denial. Denial is a mechanism we employ to protect us from a truth too painful to face. For many addicts, the truth of what it takes to maintain abstinence is too uncomfortable to tolerate. The AA program requires a person to look squarely at themselves. But for those who are constitutionally incapable of being rigorously honest, denial becomes a wall that will not allow them to look into themselves for fear of the truth they will find. For many people, the pain of abstinence becomes so severe that it blocks the ability to do the work of recovery. Sometimes we hear that pain is the great motivator, and that is true. Pain *does* motivate us to do whatever we need to do to get rid of it. It does *not* motivate us to do what will create more pain. And, when the pain of abstinence is severe and doesn't let up, it is not a motivation to stick with the painful tasks required. Rather, it interferes with the ability to do so.

Consider for a moment that you have a severe migraine headache. Or if you have never had one or know what they feel like, remember a time when you had some other severe pain. Now consider your reaction if someone were to ask you, at the point of this severe pain, to take a piece of paper and write down your character defects. How capable would you be of doing that while experiencing this pain?

But supposing you were somehow able to do that, and, after you did it, you were given another piece of paper and asked to make a list of all the people you have harmed in your life and to state what you are willing to do to make amends to these people. You would probably be constitutionally incapable of doing that. But in some drug treatment programs this is exactly what you are asked to do. These symptoms persist even with participation in recovery activities; and deep inside, the addicted person is always aware of what will provide pain relief. While some people hang on in spite of the discomfort, white knuckling it through life, many cannot and eventually give in to the compulsion to drink or take other drugs or to develop a substitute addiction such as gambling or a food addiction. *For some people, it is the pain of abstinence that renders them constitutionally incapable of being rigorously honest.*

There is currently enough scientific information about the biochemical nature of addiction to go beyond treatment methods commonly available. Traditional psychological, spiritual, and behavioral methods are helpful and should not be discarded, but it is time for a marriage between these methods and new strategies based on scientific information available. It is time to close the gap between what we know and what we do to heal the addicted brain. And that is why we have written this book.

CHAPTER 4

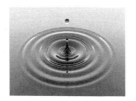

Those Amazing Amino Acids

IN OUR SEARCH FOR LASTING AND EFFECTIVE treatment for addiction, by far the most remarkable discovery so far has been amino acid therapy. Neurotransmitters are made from amino acids, the building blocks of protein. Several key neurotransmitters are particularly affected by and involved in addiction. These neurochemicals need to be balanced to their normal state in order for the recovering person to be free of abstinence symptoms such as cravings, anxiety, irritability, and depression. Over the last twenty years, numerous addiction clinicians have begun treating the brain with certain amino acids that can help restore healthy brain chemistry.

The Brain and Amino Acids

Every living cell is produced in large part from amino acids. Reproducing, altering, or growing any type of cell requires a balance of the various amino acids. Human behavior—cognition, concentration, memory, mood, sleep, thirst, appetite, alertness, and emotions—involves functioning of the whole nervous system. The nervous system is regulated almost entirely by amino acids and their biochemical companions, vitamins and minerals.

As we mentioned earlier, *neurotransmitters are produced from amino acids*: Serotonin is produced from L-tryptophan; dopamine and norepinephrine are produced from L-phenylalanine and L-tyrosine; endorphin and enkephalin levels are increased by D-phenylalanine and glutathione (composed of three amino acids—glutamic acid, glycine, and cysteine).

Amino acids and brain functioning go hand in hand. Amino acids fill the receptors of the brain and nourish it with what should be there. Neurotransmitter balance—and imbalance—is related to amino acids; neurotransmitter depletion or repletion is related to amino acids. So, in a way, it is a no-brainer (or go-brainer): restore neurotransmitters and neuroreceptors to their normal state with amino acids.

While it has become obvious that we can nourish an impoverished brain with amino acids, it is not quite as easy as it sounds. This is because the interaction of neurotransmitters is very complex with different amino acids and combinations of amino acids with their corresponding cofactors producing different effects. But still, it is fairly easy to apply. It is not a gimmick. It isn't a theory. It has been researched and been found effective in the management of addiction recovery. It works.

As we explained in earlier chapters, drug craving and chronic abstinence symptoms are a result of malfunctions of the reward centers of the brain involving the neurotransmitters and the enzymes that control them. We now know, as a result of studies done with amino acids, that it is possible to reduce stress, reduce depression, increase glucose and neurotransmitter receptor sensitivity, and restore proper levels of serotonin, dopamine, enkephalins, taurine, and GABA with amino acid supplementation.[1] If this sounds too good to be true or a dream for the future, let us assure you that it is already happening.

Essential and Nonessential Amino Acids

Amino acids are the building blocks of proteins, combining into tens of thousands of complex protein or amino acid chains of differing links and complexities called polypeptides. For example, human growth hormone is a chain of 191 amino acid molecules, while glutathione is a short chain of only three amino acids.

It is generally agreed that twenty amino acids (or twenty-one if you include L-taurine, which we do) are necessary for the creation of protein in the body. (Note: There are over 700 non-protein amino acids, which will not be discussed in this book.) Your body is able to produce many of these twenty-one amino acids from other amino acids already in the body. Because the body normally manufactures them—and hence they do not have to be in foods we eat or supplements we take—these are called nonessential amino acids. It is important to keep in mind that nonessential does not mean these amino acids are unimportant. It simply means that, under ideal circumstances, it is not essential to consume them in food or supplements.

But the body does not manufacture all of the amino acids needed in the formation of neurotransmitters. Many are derived from food sources and come to the brain by way of the blood supply. These are called essential amino acids, and, in addition to getting them from the food you eat, they can be taken as individual supplements or a formulated compound, or they can be given intravenously.

Recent scientific evidence has identified an important third category, conditionally essential amino acids. These are amino acids that are nonessential during periods free from illness and excessive stress. But during periods of illness or chronic stress (injury, surgery, excessive physical exertion, cancer therapy, or addiction) these amino acids become essential. The body's machinery is simply unable to generate adequate levels; therefore additional sources are required either from food or from supplements.

Forms of Amino Acids

Most amino acids, except glycine and taurine, can appear in two forms, the chemical structure of one being the mirror image of the other. These are called the D- and L- forms. The *D* stands for *dextro* (Latin for "right") and *L* for *levo* (Latin for "left"). These designations specify the direction of the rotation of the molecule's structural spiral as well as the direction in which light bends when passing through a liquid containing the amino acid. Products containing the L- form by far are more common in nature and more compatible with human biochemistry. All of the amino acids recommended in this book for the management of addiction are the L- form, with one important exception: D-phenylalanine.

The brain's neurotransmitters are mostly made from the chemical binding of different individual amino acids—with a few exceptions. Some individual amino acids do not have to bind with other amino acids to function as neurotransmitters; they are already neurotransmitters and do not have to be synthesized from other amino acids. Glycine, GABA, and taurine are examples of amino acids that are already neurotransmitters.

Amino Acids Related to Addiction

The following amino acids help produce the neurotransmitters most often involved in addiction:

- D-phenylalanine (increases enkephalin)
- L-phenylalanine (increases dopamine and norepinephrine)
- L-tryptophan and 5-hydroxytryptophan (5-HTP) (increases serotonin and melatonin)
- L-tyrosine (increases dopamine and norepinephrine)
- L-glutamine (increases GABA and glutathione)
- GABA (already a neurotransmitter)
- Taurine (already a neurotransmitter)

Read this list again. If you are struggling with abstinence symptoms or chronic relapse, it is of utmost importance for you to become familiar with these amino acids and what they do. The more you understand the action of amino acids and the neu-

Table 1: Essential and Nonessential Amino Acids[2]

ESSENTIAL AMINO ACIDS	NONESSENTIAL AMINO ACIDS
Isoleucine	Arginine*
Leucine	Cystine*
Lysine	Glutamine*
Methionine	Glycine
Phenylalanine	Tyrosine*
Threonine	Alanine
Tryptophan	Proline
Valine	Aspartic Acid
Histidine**	Serine
	Cystine
	Taurine*
	Glutamic Acid

* Conditionally essential amino acids
**The amino acid histidine is essential only in children.

rotransmitters they create, the better able you will be to manage your own intake and optimize your own brain neurochemistry.

Phenylalanine[3]

L-phenylalanine is an essential amino acid: that is, it must be obtained frequently from the diet in adequate quantities to meet the body's needs. Once in the brain, it can be converted into another amino acid, L-tyrosine, which in turn is used to synthesize (with the help of the cofactor vitamin B6) two key neurotransmitters, dopamine and norepinephrine.

Because of its relationship to the action of the central nervous system, L-phenylalanine can elevate mood, increase confidence and motivation, increase energy, improve alertness and wakefulness, decrease pain, indirectly decrease cravings, aid in memory and learning, and suppress the appetite.

Phenylalanine is available in three different forms: D-, L-, and DL-. (DL- is a combination of D- and L- and can be purchased as DLPA.) L-phenylalanine (LPA) is the most common type (found in nature and in food) and is the form in which phenylalanine is incorporated into the body's proteins. D-phenylalanine (DPA) increases the availability of enkephalin by inhibiting an enzyme that breaks down enkephalin, making more of it available at the reward sites in the brain. Enkephalin is a natural, morphine-like pain reliever produced by the brain, the spinal cord, and the adrenal glands. It also helps prevent pain, and produces a feeling of pleasure, even euphoria. Enkephalin also reduces stress and maintains motivation. Increased levels of enkephalin moderate or reduce alcohol consumption, while depletion or insufficiency is associated with alcohol addiction, chronic abstinence symptoms, and relapse.

Caution: Do not take L-phenylalanine if you are pregnant or nursing. Do not take it if you suffer from panic attacks or severe anxiety, both of which may be aggravated by adrenaline, derived from L-phenylalanine. Do not take it if you suffer from skin cancer melanoma or phenylketonuria (PKU). Do not use it if you are taking monoamine oxidase inhibitors (MAOIs). L-phenylalanine has been reported to cause hypertension in some people.

L-Tryptophan[4]

L-tryptophan increases the production of the neurotransmitters serotonin and melatonin which reduce cravings and help you relax and sleep. When tryptophan intake is deficient, serotonin levels drop, causing depression, anxiety, insecurity, irritability, insomnia, and lowered pain threshold. These internal conditions may result in such external behaviors as alcohol or drug abuse, carbohydrate bingeing, hyperactivity, rage, violence, sexual promiscuity, or uncontrolled gambling.

Only a few foods contain high amounts of tryptophan; most foods contain more tyrosine, which competes with tryptophan to enter the brain. Both tryptophan and 5-HTP are safe natural relaxants, tranquilizers, antidepressants, and sleep aids. When supplementing with either, it is important to also include vitamin B6, an essential cofactor in the conversion of both to serotonin.

L-Tyrosine[5]

L-tyrosine is an amino acid that helps you feel more alert and more energetic. It does this by increasing brain levels of the excitatory neurotransmitters, dopamine and norepinephrine. L-tyrosine is also an important building block for thyroid hormone. If you need a physical, mental, or emotional lift, tyrosine is the best amino acid to take. If you have any condition that makes concentration difficult, try some tyrosine and its cofactor vitamin B6.

L-Glutamine[6]

L-glutamine is an anti-craving amino acid. Whatever you crave—whether it is food, alcohol, or cocaine—glutamine will reduce the craving and help you feel more satisfied and content by directly increasing brain levels of GABA and indirectly increasing levels of enkephalins.

As a bonus, L-glutamine is the primary fuel for the inside lining of the small intestine, rapidly healing a leaky gut while protecting against damage from alcohol, aspirin, and aspirin substitutes like ibuprofen. L-glutamine is also an important precursor of the body's most powerful detoxifying and antioxidant enzyme, glutathione.

There is a lot of glutamine in uncooked animal protein, but food is not a good source of glutamine; up to 95 percent of the natural L-glutamine is inactivated by heating. The best source is a powdered supplement. It is tasteless and mixes easily with liquid (which should be cool) and is generally nontoxic. However, people with liver or kidney failure should not take L-glutamine.

GABA[7]

GABA (gamma aminobutyric acid) is both an amino acid and a neurotransmitter. GABA is the calming amino acid; it alleviates anxiety and provides a mental and physical lift. As stated earlier, glutamine works as an anti-craving substance because it stimulates production of the neurotransmitter GABA, which often becomes deficient in alcoholics and benzodiazepine addicts. Although the scientific literature states that GABA does not pass through the blood brain barrier into the brain very well, reports from recovering addicts suggest otherwise. You can take GABA or you can take L-glutamine to stimulate the production of GABA. Some people take both GABA and L-glutamine.

L-Taurine[8]

An inhibitory, calming neurotransmitter often found deficient in people with alcoholism, L-taurine is normally derived from the

metabolism of homocysteine and L-cysteine. 7
ditionally essential amino acid, and supplemer
during periods of chronic stress or illness.

Among many of its benefits, L-taurine acts as a brain, liver, and heart cell antioxidant, by scavenging excess free radicals. It also serves as a neurotransmitter, joining with cholesterol to form an important component of bile. It helps regulate intracellular concentrations of magnesium, calcium, potassium, and sodium.

David: I had maintained more than ten years of abstinence from alcohol when I first heard of amino acid therapy. While I had learned to cope with the discomfort of sobriety, I had found nothing that truly gave me relief. I still struggled with stimulus augmentation and stress sensitivity. Another addiction professional told me about an amino acid formulation and suggested I try it. I did, more because he asked me to than because I expected a positive result. I noticed the effect almost immediately. The major benefit was the reduction in stimulus augmentation. Everything seemed toned down. Life was less shrill. I felt less bombarded by sounds and things going on around me. In a word, I felt relief. It was as if I were wrapped in a soothing blanket. My internal molecules seemed to quiet and stop fighting me. I felt at ease. It felt as if I had taken a stone out of my shoe. The effect was so dramatic that Merlene noticed it right away. She said I seemed more relaxed and easy to be around. In fact, over time I discovered that any time I failed to take the amino acid supplement she would say, "Did you take your nutrients?" sometimes before even I realized that I had forgotten. I realize now that for the first time in my life I was functioning at a comfort level that seemed to begin in my brain, filtered throughout my body, and affected my behavior. Even though I still had some ups and downs with mood, this level of comfort became my normal state, and the ups and downs are much easier to deal with.

Some Background

One person who has done extensive work with amino acid therapy is our colleague, Julia Ross (author of *The Diet Cure*[9] and *The Mood Cure*[10]), director of Recovery Systems in Mill Valley, California. Julia has been using oral amino acid supplementation and dietary nutrition to modify brain chemistry with tremendous reported success for seventeen years. We have had the opportunity to spend time with Julia, learn from her experience and expertise, and integrate her knowledge of amino acid therapy with our experience with preventing relapse.

Julia began her use of amino acid therapy, as we did, after hearing about the work of Kenneth Blum in the 1980s. Blum, who had spent many years studying the neurochemistry of addiction, began investigating ways to alter the brain chemistry of addicted people to give them the comfort needed to participate in the recovery process. He reasoned that if the interaction of neurotransmitters does not function normally to provide a reward, then craving leads to addiction which leads to more craving which, of course, interferes with recovery.

After studying the genetics of addiction, Blum took the next logical step—correcting the neurotransmitter abnormalities with the natural substances that produce them, amino acids. He developed the first oral supplement of amino acids formulated specifically for people in recovery.

The following table describes the action of neurotransmitters most often related to addiction, the mood-altering substances that are often used when there is a deficiency, the amino acids that normally produce the neurotransmitters, and the result of a deficiency of each neurotransmitter.

Neurotransmitter	Action	Substance	Deficiency Symptoms	Amino Acids
Dopamine	Good feelings, satisfaction, comfort, alertness	Alcohol, marijuana, cocaine, caffeine, amphetamines, sugar, tobacco	"Emptiness," lack of pleasure and reward, fatigue, depression	L-phenylalanine, L-tyrosine
Norepinepherine	Arousal, energy, stimulation, mental focus	Cocaine, speed tobacco, sugar, marijuana, alcohol	Lack of energy, depression, poor concentration	L-phenylalanine, L-tyrosine
GABA	Calming, relaxation	Valium, alcohol, tobacco, marijuana	Anxiety, panic, insecurity, insomnia	GABA, L-glutamine
Endorphins/ Enkephalins	Physical and emotional pain relief, pleasure, good feelings, euphoria	Heroin, alcohol, marijuana, sugar, chocolate	Hypersensitivity to emotional/physical pain, anhedonia, cravings, incompleteness, "blahs"	D-phenylalanine, DL-phenylalanine
Serotonin	Emotional stability, self-confidence, pain tolerance	Alcohol, sugar, chocolate, tobacco, marijuana	Depression, worry, low self-esteem, fearfulness, obsessiveness, violence, compulsiveness, tantrums	L-tryptophan, 5-HTP
Taurine	Calmness, promotion of sleep and digestion, seizure control	Benzodiazepines, alcohol	Proneness to seizures, sleeplessness, anxiety, poor digestion	Taurine

Scientific Studies

In the 1950s, Dr. Roger Williams, a pioneer in the study of alcoholism and nutrition, discovered that taking 3,000 to 4,000 mg (one rounded teaspoon) of glutamine daily would stop alcohol cravings and decrease cravings for sweets.[11]

Through double-blind studies, we now know that amino acid supplementation can reduce drug hunger (craving), reduce stress, reduce or eliminate withdrawal tremors, reduce cocaine-induced dreams, increase libido, reduce physiological stress, improve behavior, increase focus, increase glucose receptor sensitivity, and restore neurotransmitters such as serotonin, dopamine, enkephalins, taurine, and GABA.

Studies on an amino acid supplement formulated specifically for alcoholics[12] showed that the supplement users experienced significantly less stress, drug craving, depression, irritability, paranoia, anger, and anxiety. They also had more energy, self-confidence, and feelings of well-being. They were six times more likely to complete a twenty-eight-day treatment program and had fewer incidents of relapse.

Studies on an amino acid supplement formulated for stimulant abusers[13] have established that the supplement users had a 50 percent lower drug hunger score than the control group. They also had a treatment dropout rate of 4.6 percent, compared to 37 percent for the control group and a relapse rate of 20 percent, compared to 87 percent for the control group.

For carbohydrate bingers,[14] those who took the amino acid supplement for ninety days lost an average of twenty-seven pounds and had a relapse rate of 18 percent. Those in the control group lost an average of ten pounds, with a relapse rate of 82 percent.

In a study published in 1997, two groups of dieters were monitored for two years after completing a medically monitored fast. During the fast, the dieters used a powdered nutri-

Tryptophan for Depression

Two researchers in England compared the effects of tryptophan and the popular prescription drug Tofranil. (Tofranil, or imipramine, is a commonly used antidepressant.) Both groups of patients with depression improved. The study revealed that tryptophan was just as effective as Tofranil, and there were no side effects from the tryptophan. Conversely, the side effects for the Tofranil group included blurring of vision, dryness of mouth, low blood pressure, urinary retention, heart palpitations, hepatitis, and seizures.

From *Heal with Amino Acids and Nutrients*[12]

tional drink (Optifast) in place of two or three meals each day. (It is now well recognized that liquid dieters can lose weight rapidly but soon regain it when they go off the liquid diet. This is because the body has gone into starvation mode; when food is available again, the body stores it for future periods of starvation.) In this study, after completing the fast, one group took an amino acid formulation each day, and the other group did not. At the end of two years, the amino acid group showed:

- A twofold decrease in percent overweight for both males and females.
- A 70 percent decrease in cravings for females and a 63 percent decrease in cravings for males.
- A 66 percent decrease in binge eating for females and a 41 percent decrease for males.
- Only a 14.7 percent regain of weight lost while the control group regained 41.7 percent of their lost weight.

The Blood-Brain Barrier

Nutrients are carried throughout the body via the bloodstream. As these nutrients pass by, each organ reaches out and takes what it needs to maintain itself. Since there are substances in the bloodstream that can injure the brain, it is surrounded by a paper-thin, highly selective, protective membrane that is difficult to penetrate. Certain proteins called transporter or carrier proteins move through the barrier and expedite the passage of select nutrients into the brain. But if too many amino acids seek to cross into the brain at one time, the transporters become overloaded and only the amino acids in greatest supply are allowed in.

This is why you are advised to take amino acid supplements on an empty stomach—to avoid making them compete for absorption with the amino acids in food. If you take an amino acid supplement with a high-protein meal, the ones you need most may not be the ones to penetrate the blood-brain barrier. It is best to take individual amino acids between meals with small amounts of vitamin B6 and vitamin C to enhance absorption.

If you are taking more than one amino acid, you may want to take them at different times of day. Take L-tyrosine, for instance, when you want to be alert and focused, and take tryptophan when you want to relax or go to sleep. If you are taking a formulation of amino acids, you may want to supplement the formulation at a different time of day with an amino acid for which you have a specific need.

Oral Amino Acid Therapy

Deficiencies of certain amino acids may predispose people to use stimulant drugs, other deficiencies may lead to use of calming drugs, while other deficiencies will lead to use of pain killers. Likewise, excessive use of different drugs will cause or intensify different deficiencies (e.g., alcohol abuse results in poor absorption of L-tryptophan from the blood into the brain, resulting in a deficiency of serotonin). The symptoms experienced with abstinence will depend on what conditions existed before the use of substances, what drugs have been used and how heavily those drugs were used.

Rather than determining which amino acids are appropriate based on what drug has been used, however, it may be more appropriate to determine what effect you get from the drug, and even more on what symptoms are experienced when the drug is *not* used. The following table offers some helpful guidelines:

Table 2: Guidelines for Choosing Amino Acids

Abstinence Symptoms	Suggested Amino Acids
anxiety, stress, tension	GABA, taurine, 5-HTP
low energy, apathy	L-tyrosine
poor concentration, poor memory, mental fuzziness	L-tyrosine
hypersensitivity	L-phenylalanine, D-phenylalanine
sleeplessness	L-tryptophan or 5 HTP, GABA, taurine
irritability, negativity, worry	L-tryptophan or 5-HTP
cravings	L-glutamine, GABA, L-tryptophan, 5-HTP
depression, anhedonia	L-tyrosine

The minimum effective starting dose for most amino acids is 100 mg per day. This can be gradually increased to 3,000 mg per day (except for 5-HTP, which ranges in dosage from 50 to 300 mg per day, and L-glutamine, which ranges in dosage from 250 to 12,000 mg per day) until the desired benefits are observed. Most people respond to daily doses of 500 to 1,500 mg in divided dosages two to three times per day. Amino acids are most effective when taken with water on an empty stomach, especially the larger amino acids (phenylalanine, tryptophan, and 5-HTP) that compete with each other for access to the brain from the bloodstream.

If you are taking any medications, you should only use these amino acids under medical supervision. Do not use them if you are taking MAO inhibitors (MAOIs) or any drugs that affect the particular brain chemicals listed in the table on page 77. Always read the labels and never take anything that is contraindicated for any condition you may have.

Always take amino acids with a good multivitamin/mineral supplement. They are important for their individual roles, but also because they help the amino acids make it to the brain and aid in conversion of amino acids into neurotransmitters. In creating brain neurotransmitters, amino acids rarely act alone. With the exception of individual free amino acids that are already neurotransmitters (e.g., taurine and glycine), amino acids need the help of vitamins and minerals (cofactors) before the formation can take place. For example, vitamin B6 is needed to manufacture dopamine and serotonin, and vitamin C helps convert dopamine to norepinephrine.

Rebalancing brain chemistry is not just a matter of taking a certain amino acid to produce serotonin, a different one to produce dopamine, or yet another to raise opioid levels. As we have stated previously, neurotransmitters interact in a pattern of stimulation and inhibition to bring about a neurochemical reward. Dopamine has been identified as the primary neurotransmitter associated with addiction, but it never works in isolation. It is the interaction of the various neurotransmitters that brings about a dopamine reward in the limbic system of the brain and reduces symptoms of reward deficiency and abstinence. Although a single amino acid may be involved in the formation of a given neurotransmitter, it may require a combination or formulation to correct the problem.

"No drug currently in wide use, medical or recreational, addresses the root cause of neurotransmitter levels. Drugs merely stimulate temporary excessive release of pre-existing neurotransmitter stores. They do not increase production of neurotransmitters. . . . Greater transport into the brain of the relevant amino acids vitamins, and minerals augment nourishment of the brain when there are less than adequate levels."

Heal with Amino Acids and Nutrients[16]

Supplements that Support Amino Acid Therapy

Amino acid supplements alone are not effective. They need help from other nutrients. Following are supplements that we recommend to provide additional nourishment for the brain or to activate or synergize the amino acids.

Pyridoxal-5-phosphate (P-5-P) is the activated form of vitamin B6. Some people are unable to activate B6 (perhaps because they are deficient in zinc or riboflavin). Pyridoxal-5-phosphate is an important cofactor in the production of dopamine (and hence norepinephrine) and also serotonin (and hence melatonin).

NADH is a natural chemical in the body capable of stimulating enzymes to manufacture dopamine and, to a lesser degree, serotonin. NADH has been clinically shown to reverse mild to moderate depression and to help prevent and reverse symptoms of ADHD. It is also a powerful brain-protecting antioxidant.

Folate, or folic acid, lowers homocysteine levels and raises SAMe and key neurotransmitter levels. According to Abram Hoffer, MD, at very high doses (5,000 to 25,000 mcg daily), folate is a highly effective antidepressant. A more effective form of folate may be methyl folate, its active form in the human body.

Methylcobalamin is the active form of vitamin B12. Studies indicate that it's more effective and better absorbed orally than the customary cyanocobalamin or hydroxycobalamin.

Magnesium taurate is chelated magnesium (magnesium chemically bound to an amino acid) and is better absorbed and a more effective form of magnesium. Early studies that combined magnesium to taurine indicate a superior ability to control seizures, lower blood pressure, protect the heart, and induce sleep.

Zinc is an important nutrient because a deficiency is associated with a myriad of conditions, including those associated with addiction and substance abuse. These conditions include: hyperactivity; poor attention span; poor healing from wounds, injuries, and infections; chronic diarrhea; anorexia; elevated homocysteine blood levels (hence an increased risk of heart attacks, cancer, and strokes, as well as low brain levels of glutathione, SAMe, melatonin, serotonin, and norepinephrine); low vitamin A levels; learning disorders/impaired learning; poor memory; delinquent behavior; aggression; adrenal insufficiency; immune deficiency; HIV/AIDS; alcoholism (a large amount of zinc is lost in urine); and clinical depression.

Safety

Since the inception of amino acid therapy in the mid-1980s thousands of people have taken them safely with few side effects. There have been almost no complaints to the FDA regarding their use. The one exception was a contamination problem with L-tryptophan in 1988. One batch manufactured in Japan was contaminated and went untested, causing 1,500 people to become ill, resulting in thirty-seven deaths. It was not the L-tryptophan itself that was the problem but a new processing method that resulted in contamination.

Why Food Is Not Enough

Since the primary source of amino acids is food, you may be asking if a deficiency can be resolved with diet alone. The answer is: maybe, but not likely. Certainly, foods are important and we will discuss that in another chapter. You can get L-tryptophan from milk to produce serotonin. You can eat meat or eggs for tyrosine to produce dopamine. And these will help you. But diet alone is probably not enough to fix deficiencies—for several reasons.

Modern farming, food processing, and cooking practices result in foods that may not provide the nutrition that our brains need. For example, up to 95 percent of L-glutamine is destroyed by cooking. In addition, many people have food allergies and may not digest and absorb nutrients well. The result is amino acid deficiency. Add to that the fact that you may have a genetic condition, aggravated by addiction and stress, that has created a need for higher levels of amino acids than you can get from diet alone.

There is a catch-22 in attempting to control craving with diet. In the absence of your drug of choice, there is often a serotonin insufficiency and a resulting overwhelming craving for carbohydrates. The cravings interfere with the ability to maintain a proper nutritional plan long enough to overcome the cravings. Amino acid supplements can offset these cravings rather quickly to support other changes in your diet.

No Magic Bullet

We do not want to give you the impression that amino acid therapy is a cure-all. There isn't one. While we are raving fans of amino acid supplementation, it is not a substitute for good nutrition or other aspects of healthful living. (That's why it's called supplementation, not substitution.) Nor do we want you to believe that everyone who takes an amino acid product and will get an immediate result as David did. Many do, and you may also; or, you may need to experiment a little. For instance, if you try GABA to help you relax and sleep better, yet don't get the result you are seeking, try tryptophan and taurine instead.

Occasionally people do have mild side effects or an unusual reaction such as an upset stomach, especially with large doses of amino acids. In these instances no permanent harm will be done as the amino acids leave the body within one to four hours. If this should happen to you and you are taking multiple amino acids, stop taking all of them and reintroduce them one by one until you can determine which one is causing the problem. Sometimes if the reaction is mild you might want to persist in taking it to see if the situation gradually improves. Frequently the reaction occurs only in the first few days as the body adjusts. The benefits may prove to be well worth the persistence.

Sometimes you may experience undesired results because of taking the wrong amino acid. Finding the right amino acids or combination of amino acids for you is not an exact science and may require some experimentation on your part. Please do not give up if you do not attain the desired response immediately.

An Amino Acid Complex

You can buy amino acids individually at a pharmacy or a health food store. But for some people, especially recovering addicts who may feel overwhelmed by all they have to do to stay sober, remembering to take the appropriate amino acid at the right time of day (up to six capsules or tablets of each amino acid, two or three at a time) may become more than they can manage. For them compounded formulations of amino acids are available. Each tablet or capsule contains several amino acids, making it unnecessary to take each one separately. (Remember, however, that while this may be easier, you will be less able to adjust what you take to your individual needs.) Another option is to get nutrients in packets of what you need to take at one time. These are available from LifeStream Solutions at http://www.lifestream-solutions.com.

Compounded amino acid products or packets are available in different formulations. The formulation you should select depends largely on your drug of choice and on what produces the optimum effect for you. If you prefer drugs like alcohol or heroin that depress the nervous system, you will probably get the best result from a formulation that will help you relax, developed for people who prefer downers. If you prefer drugs like cocaine or methamphetamine, you will more likely benefit from a formulation developed for people who have used uppers to give you a lift and help you be more alert. See Appendix C for questionnaires to help you determine what nutrients are most likely best for you.

Just as it is with individual amino acids, it is best to take a formulation or nutrients in packets thirty to sixty minutes before or one to two hours after a meal. At a different time of day, some people supplement this with the amino acid they need most. Carol, a recovering alcoholic who also has attention deficit disorder, has found that if she takes a formulation of phenylalanine, tyrosine, glutamine, and important vitamin and mineral cofactors twice a day, she still has a down time in the afternoon when she has difficulty concentrating and feels slightly irritable. Some additional tyrosine in the afternoon gives her a lift, improving her mood, alertness, and concentration. Trial and error will probably result in the reward you are seeking.

Guidelines for Amino Acid Supplementation

Here are some guidelines to maximize the benefits of amino acid supplementation and minimize any adverse reactions:

- Take amino acids on an empty stomach, ideally thirty minutes or more before or at least an hour after meals containing protein. Protein is made up of amino acids and some of these will compete with and crowd out those you are taking. If you absolutely cannot remember to take the supplements on an empty stomach, increase the dose. Amino acids will still help you but not as much as they will if you take them on an empty stomach. An exception to this is tryptophan. If you take tryptophan with protein, you will probably not get any benefit from it. Take it alone or with a carbohydrate, no-protein snack.
- If you have sleep problems, don't take tyrosine or phenylalanine after 2:00 p.m.
- If you become jittery, wired, or hyper, stop taking tyrosine or phenylalanine. Take the inhibitory, calming glutamine, taurine, or GABA to reverse the effects. If that is not enough, take tryptophan (always on an empty stomach).

- If you become too relaxed or spacey, stop taking GABA, taurine, glutamine, or tryptophan. Take tyrosine to counteract the effects.
- If you get a headache take chelated magnesium, vitamin B, and vitamin C.
- If you don't get the benefits you are seeking from the appropriate amino acid, gradually increase the dose to the maximum recommended.
- Often SAMe (S-adenosyl methionine, 800 to 1,600 mg a day in individual doses) will help your brain better utilize the amino acids. Although it usually starts working within a few days, try it for at least a week because it can take that long to feel the effects. Since SAMe is derived from the proper metabolism of homocysteine, lowering homocysteine with therapeutic levels of B12 and B6 results in increased SAMe levels.
- Sometimes oral supplements don't work because of poor absorption or other factors. In that case, we strongly suggest that you (1) pursue medical care to heal the condition that is interfering with getting adequate nutrition, (2) read *Mood Cure* by Julia Ross for a more in-depth understanding of what may be your problem, (3) seriously consider bypassing the digestive tract with intravenous nutritional therapy, which will be discussed in the next chapter.
- Remember that anyone taking amino acids must take vitamin B6 to properly metabolize them. If you are insufficiently nourished with vitamin B6, all the amino acids in the world will not produce adequate amounts of the neurotransmitters your brain hungers for.
- When you are especially stressed, you may want to take more than your normal dose.

Experts do not agree on how long a recovering person needs to take amino acid supplements. People with less severe addictions may be able to discontinue daily amino acid supplements after a relatively short period of time. But chronic relapsers, those with pre-existing conditions such as ADHD, and people who continue to be uncomfortable when abstinent need all the help they can get, probably for life. This means giving the brain—daily—what it cannot produce naturally with a combination of nutritious food and amino acid supplements.

You will be surprised at how much better you will feel when you take the right amino acids at the right dosage for you. You will not feel high. You will just feel more normal—happier and less irritable, more calm, rested, and alert. In addition you will have noticeably fewer drug and carbohydrate cravings.

If for any reason you are unable to take amino acid supplements, you might have to consider other ways of getting the needed amino acids. For some people they do not work because they are not absorbed, and a few people experience mild nausea. If you decide the supplements are not right for you, you may want to consider getting a periodic intravenous amino acid booster. If not, remember that amino acids come from food. If you do not take the supplements, it is important to pay closer attention to what you eat and when. But that is also important even if you do take the supplements.

Thanks to Dr. James Braly and Julia Ross for help in writing this chapter. For information about programs using amino acid and vitamin therapy, contact us at LifeStream Solutions at 1-800-287-0906.

CHAPTER 5

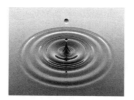

Intravenous Delivery of
Mood-Boosting Nutrients

IT SEEMED LIKE A MIRACLE when we came across it several years ago. And it still is, by far, the most successful treatment for addiction that we have come across anywhere—intravenous delivery of brain-healing nutrients. With this method of delivery there is immediate relief from chronic abstinence symptoms, and an immediate reduction in the severity of symptoms that usually take weeks or months to diminish. Brain chemistry is rebalanced with rapid relief from cravings. Recovery is accelerated, and physical, mental, and emotional symptoms are reversed. This therapy provides a jump-start for recovery that allows people to better participate in the other aspects of addiction treatment and to do so with more clarity and optimism. It improves the quality and comfort of sobriety and reduces the risk of relapse.

LifeStream Follow-up Study

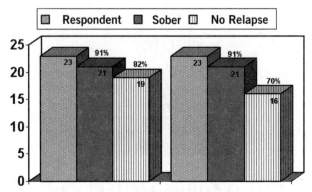

In a small follow-up study of clients who received nutritional therapy using diet, supplements, and intravenous treatment at Bridging the Gaps in Winchester, Virginia, of twenty-three respondents having one to two years since treatment:

- 91 percent were sober at six months with 82% having no relapse
- 91 percent were sober at the time of contact with 70 percent having no relapse

Numerous treatment centers in the United States are now delivering amino acids, vitamins, and minerals intravenously to provide a recovery jump-start and to allow nutrients to enter the brain in larger quantities than is possible orally. The intravenous process overcomes many of the problems that exist with taking amino acid products by mouth. The effectiveness of the oral supplements is limited to the few hours around the time they are taken, whereas intravenous delivery has an ongoing effect long after the treatment ceases.

Another advantage to the intravenous liquid solution is that it does not have to go through the gastrointestinal absorption process. People absorb nutrients from the intestinal tract in different quantities and at different rates. One person might absorb 98 percent of the amino acids taken by mouth, while another person may only absorb 8 percent. There is no way to monitor this to determine the appropriate dosage. So it is impossible to know how much of what goes into the mouth is actually absorbed into and utilized by the brain. In addition, addicted people have often damaged their bodies with their alcohol or other drug use to the extent that they have leaky gut syndrome, which means they absorb little of what they consume (and, therefore, absorb little of the amino acids and vitamins they take in). With intravenous delivery, the digestive tract is bypassed, and the body utilizes all the nutrients delivered. It should be pointed out here that many people who come for intravenous treatment come as a last resort. They are not addicts in early or middle-stage addiction or those who are easy to treat. They may have failed at multiple attempts at recovery in the past and are willing to try this therapy only because they have no other options. They may have lost all hope of being able to attain, let alone maintain, sobriety. We point this out to make it clear that intravenous nutritional therapy is not just successful for people who are highly motivated or less sick than people who go through other treatment programs. No—the fact is that in many cases they are sicker, more hopeless, and more difficult to treat, with a long history of relapse. We recommend it for anyone who wants to get a head start on recovery and feel better in just a few days than they would otherwise feel weeks into sobriety.

Intravenous treatment can be given for detoxification, or it can be given directly after medical detoxification or for enhancing the quality of ongoing recovery.

Intravenous Nutritional Detox

The first few days of intravenous nutritional detoxification may be a little uncomfortable, but it's nothing like what addicts have experienced with other types of detox. For many people, the detoxification process is so uncomfortable that they never make it all the way through. Which means they never get to the rehabilitation part of treatment. Eric was one of those people. He told his counselor before beginning intravenous nutritional detox that he had never made it more than three days in a detox program despite having tried numerous methods. People who knew Eric jokingly called this his three-day syndrome. He said when he began intravenous nutritional therapy that if he was still there on day four it would mean something was working. For the first couple of days, Eric was mildly uncomfortable, had trouble sleeping, and was a bit irritable. But the therapy was far from intolerable, and he did not think of leaving. By day three, he was feeling good, sleeping, and was very hopeful. On day four, he told his counselor that his three-day-syndrome was history. Eric had not only made it through the detoxification period but was already experiencing clarity of thought that typically does not come with conventional treatment, even at the end of a twenty-eight-day program.

Following the IV detox, Eric went on to further treatment, which had never been possible before. Eric's symptoms, even during the first couple of days, were far less severe than those he experienced with other forms of detox. No matter how effective a treatment program is in helping a person adjust to sobriety and develop the skills for living sober, it can't help a person who finds withdrawal so painful that he or she leaves before ever getting the toxic substance out of the body. Treatment program recovery rates seldom include the people who leave before they completely detox.

But first let's talk about what usually happens in conventional treatment as people go through social or medical detoxification. Social detox generally takes place outside of a medical setting and is done cold turkey (no medication). Detoxing cold turkey can be very painful, and it's also dangerous. Seizures, hallucinations, and even death can occur. (With intravenous nutritional detoxification, none of these serious problems are known to have occurred.) If a person in a social detox program shows signs of severe distress (such as having a seizure), the patient is taken to a medical facility for medical detoxification.

Some people don't take the risk of undergoing a social detox program. This is advisable, especially if the drug from which they are withdrawing is a depressant such as alcohol or heroin. During medical detoxification, a drug chemically similar to the one being removed from the body is given to ease the severity of withdrawal symptoms. The dose is gradually reduced as symptoms subside. For example, Librium or Valium are often used to detox someone from alcohol, because these drugs calm the nervous system and allow the body to gradually adjust to the absence of alcohol. During this process, the patient can still experience severe discomfort and tremors, nausea, vomiting, and occasionally even delirium tremens (DTs).

Medical detox is much safer than social detox, of course. However, it takes longer than the IV nutritional process because the addicted person also has to withdraw from the substitute drug. With IV nutritional detoxification no substitute medication is necessary, so the process is faster. Patients treated with intravenous amino acids and vitamins report that withdrawal symptoms are mild enough that there is no need to use any medication.

We should point out here that it is never wise or safe to stop any kind of downer drug (alcohol, heroin, methadone, painkillers, benzodiazepines, sleep medications, or antidepressants) suddenly. As we said, sudden withdrawal can lead to seizures and can be life threatening. These drugs require gradual tapering unless one is detoxing with IV nutrients under supervision of a medical doctor.

With medical detox it is possible withdraw from alcohol or heroin in a matter of days. Drugs such as benzodiazepines (tranquilizers), sleep medications, painkillers, and antidepressants require a much slower tapering-off period. Withdrawing from antidepressants can take weeks. Withdrawing from benzodiazepines can take months. If you taper too fast, you will experience high levels of anxiety, severe insomnia, tremors, body jerks, and other symptoms that can interfere with the ability to function. If you need to taper off benzodiazepines or antidepressants, ask your doctor to use the Ashton method (http://www.geocities. com/benzobusters/manual.htm). You can taper faster if you are taking GABA. LifeStream's GABA Paks have the right amount of GABA and other nutrients you need. Our preference, if possible, is to combine a taper with weekly intravenous nutrient treatments.

With intravenous nutritional treatment for other drugs, patients notice that all craving is gone by day three or four. This is usually a surprise to them, because craving has been a part of their lives so long that they don't remember what it feels like not to have it. But they are pleased to find that they have no desire for drugs. They feel satisfied and at ease.

Around day four or five, most people are amazed by their clarity of thought. They don't have the fuzzy thinking they had with other treatments. Clay said, "I felt so mentally sharp. I had never felt like that before. I can think so clearly." Another patient who had previously experienced some fairly long periods of sobriety with the help of AA commented that his thinking was clearer after five days than it had been after a year of sobriety in the past. "I feel like I'm starting recovery with my first year behind me," he said.

There is a dramatic change in appearance, especially in the eyes. People who come to the clinic looking very ill suddenly look bright and alive. Even people who have had extended periods of sobriety in the past often say they feel better than they have ever felt in their lives.

A commonly asked question is: How long does it last? While the experts don't yet know for sure, two key ingredients in the success of intravenous amino acid therapy are already clear. First, those who have been educated about the nature of their addiction fare best; and second, individuals who have developed a self-care plan and a good relapse prevention plan also do best after IV treatment. It is becoming increasingly evident that people need education about recovery; they need to know the importance of maintaining good nutrition and healthy lifestyle, and thus, healthy brain chemistry. We know that poor nutrition or the use of nicotine or prescription drugs or even severe stress can reduce the effects of intravenous amino acid therapy. So we highly recommend that patients take amino acid and vitamin supplements daily following initial treatment. This helps them maintain the neurochemical balance that has been restored.

After intravenous nutritional therapy, patients are better able to do the other work of recovery, because their cravings are gone, their minds are clear, and they feel better. Many changes must occur to maintain sobriety, but these changes are very difficult when craving, mental confusion, and internal discomfort interfere with the ability to make these changes.

Relief from Chronic Abstinence Symptoms

Some centers don't accept clients until they are already detoxed. Intravenous therapy is still very beneficial. It is the most effective method we have found for relieving abstinence symptoms, not just those that emerge shortly after abstinence begins but also those that persist long-term.

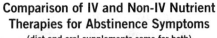

Comparison of IV and Non-IV Nutrient Therapies for Abstinence Symptoms
(diet and oral supplements same for both)

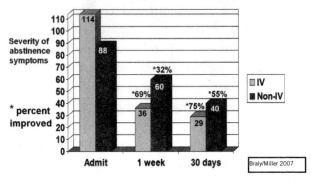

In a six-month comparison of intravenous-oral nutritional therapy to non-intravenous nutritional therapy, intravenous therapy was found to be more effective in reducing the severity of abstinence symptoms than oral nutritional therapy alone. Dr. James Braly compared two groups of clients at Bridging the Gaps in Winchester, Virginia. One group received intravenous and oral nutritional therapy and the other received oral nutritional therapy only. The Abstinence Symptom Severity Scale (see Appendix B) was used to assess the severity of symptoms in each group before the start of nutritional therapy, daily for six days, and again at thirty days. The group receiving intravenous therapy had a greater reduction in the severity of sobriety symptoms in six days than the group that received oral therapy alone had in thirty days. Diet and oral supplements were the same for both.

Many people who have maintained long-term continuous sobriety—for months or years—following traditional treatment may struggle with symptoms of impaired brain chemistry that never go away. These symptoms can quickly be relieved with intravenous nutritional therapy. Thus it can improve the quality of life for people who are no longer using drugs but who may not be comfortable in sobriety.

Bob had been sober for twelve years, still attended AA regularly, and thought that his life was as good as it was going to get. He was grateful for AA and the years of abstinence it had given him. But he was never really comfortable. He was stress-sensitive and sometimes quite irritable. He had difficulty concentrating. Mainly he just had a sense of internal discomfort that he could not describe but which never went away. He was not even close to taking a drink, but he did want to feel better.

Eventually, Bob met someone who had received intravenous nutritional treatment and he was surprised that this person could be feeling so good so early in recovery. He began to wonder if it would work for him even though he hadn't had a drink in twelve years. He decided to try it. Bob immediately found relief from the ongoing discomfort that had been with him for so long. Two years later, he is still an enthusiastic supporter of the treatment and tells anyone who will listen about a way to feel better even years after they have stopped using drugs.

Sometimes patients feel so good after IV nutritional therapy that they become overconfident about their ability to stay sober. At this point, they have no desire to drink or use, so they believe they never will. But addiction is much more than brain chemistry. It affects all areas of life. Recovering people must also learn new patterns of behavior. Their lives must change. This doesn't happen automatically just because the brain has been able to heal.

Sometimes, however, it is difficult for people who have had IV nutritional treatment to find acceptance right away in a support group. It is difficult for people who have struggled or are still struggling in sobriety to believe that someone can feel as good with only days of sobriety as intravenous amino acid patients often do.

Paul went to his first mutual help meeting shortly after

receiving IV nutritional therapy. He told the others in the group it was his first meeting and he had two weeks of sobriety. He described the kind of treatment he had and said how good he felt. Not surprisingly, the group was skeptical, telling him, "You are still on a pink cloud. You will come back down. You are in denial." One group member told him he wouldn't last two months. Paul was disappointed by this reaction to what he considered a miracle in his life. But he continued to go to meetings and he continued to feel good. That was several years ago, and he has maintained his sobriety despite the negative predictions.

You must also remember that, for the most part, we are talking about chronic relapsers—people who have relapsed over and over again with conventional treatment. As we pointed out previously, in many cases the people who come for IV treatment are not getting treatment for the first, or even the second, time. They are those who have already tried conventional treatment, and they're the ones who may not be able to receive treatment anywhere else because they have relapsed so many times before. They are the ones who have given up hope that they will ever be able to find comfortable sober living. Many do find comfort and serenity following conventional treatment. But it is for those who don't that IV treatment is truly a life-saving miracle.

A Story of Recovery: Like so many others who find that the road to recovery turns out to be a mountain to climb, Brian was a chronic heroin relapser. He doesn't remember how many times he has been in treatment—sometimes for a few days, a few times for months. One time he went in for detox and four hours later was calling his dealer. One time he stayed sober for two years. One time he stayed sober long enough to get married and have a baby. But when his wife discovered he was using heroin again, she took the baby and left. During his times of sobriety, he went to twelve-step meetings and talked about how grateful he was to be clean. He had an outgoing personality and everyone liked him. He seemed to enjoy life. But Brian had a secret. He never stopped thinking about using heroin. He told himself he only had to make it one day at a time. But every day was a little harder than the one before. He couldn't get rid of the thought that if he could just use heroin once his life would be better. He usually began using in secret and was able to keep anyone from knowing for quite a while. But eventually he would be caught; and back to treatment he would go. Clean again, but not happy, not comfortable. Everyone who had believed in him began to give up on him. He finally gave up on himself and decided there was no point in getting straight if he could never maintain it.

But Brian was fortunate. He had a friend who didn't give up on him. Joe kept encouraging Brian to try again. Joe heard about intravenous nutritional treatment and told Brian about it. It was a hard sell, but Brian agreed to give it a try. What did he have to lose? He felt that his life was over anyway. And deep in his heart he yearned to be able to live a clean and sober life. He had a lot to live for.

As part of treatment, Brian developed a plan for ongoing self care and a plan for changing his behavior if he began regressing toward relapse at any time. After receiving the IV nutritional treatment, Brian felt a sense of relief he had never experienced before. In fact, he felt even better than he had before he began using heroin. At first, Brian kept waiting for the other shoe to drop. He kept expecting the craving and the yearning for heroin to return, but it didn't. He went to outpatient treatment for some time, and it was different from how it had been in the past. He was able to think more clearly and better able to apply what he was learning to his life.

Brian cautiously began to rebuild his life. Even though he had been able to play the role of a happy sober person in the past, this time the difference was noticeable. There was something in Brian's appearance and demeanor that was new and different. He was, for the first time, comfortable without drugs. He still took life one day at a time, but instead of every day being harder than the one before, now every day was better. He wasn't able to save his marriage, but he was able to become an active parent. In his distant past he had been an artist and began to paint again. He has been clean longer than ever before. But the length of sobriety isn't as important to Brian as the quality of life. He feels he is really living now, not just holding on.

For information about programs using intravenous or oral amino acid therapy, contact us at LifeStream Solutions at 800-287-0906.

CHAPTER 6

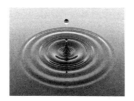

This Is Your Brain on Food

To this point we have discussed supplements that will improve the quality of sobriety and help prevent relapse. But supplements are not more important than the food you eat daily. Nutrition is one of the most important aspects of recovery. And the more we learn about the relationship of the brain to addiction and of nutrition to the functioning of the brain, the more we know that poor nutrition and problems in sobriety are very much related. In order to protect sobriety, you need a nutrition plan based on sound nutritional principles.

Whatever you do to get sober and whatever else you do to stay sober, good nutrition should be a central part of recovery. Good nutrition includes food as well as supplements. Long-term recovery from addiction requires healthful eating and an adequate supply of amino acids, vitamins, and minerals. Not for a short period of time; not just until you are feeling better; not just until the initial withdrawal and craving are gone. A person seeking freedom from the discomfort of addiction must make the same kind of commitment to healthful eating that a diabetic must make. We have no magic bullet to fix either the pancreas or the brain once and for all. Dysfunction of both requires special care on a regular basis.

However, we have to admit that good nutrition is a moving target. Just about the time we think we have it all figured out, along comes a new study that lets us know that nobody has all the answers. And then we have to find out if the new study is valid. Not all studies can be trusted completely. There is often more—or less—to the picture than we are told. Especially if the studies have been supported by an interest group that has something to gain or lose by the outcome of the study or report. And remember that you have to consider your own situation and weigh the information accordingly. For instance, it has been reported that one glass of wine a day may be good for your heart. But this is certainly not the case if you are a recovering alcoholic. One glass of wine a day may lead to several and finally a full-blown relapse—certainly not good for your heart.

So do not take the information you get here (or anywhere else for that matter) as the last word on your health. Keep an open mind and learn as much as possible about nutrition. In this chapter we are not going to talk specifically about a diet to prevent cancer, to strengthen your heart, or to help you lose weight. You will need to take these things into consideration as you make a nutrition plan for yourself. And there is plenty of information out there. We will mainly talk about nutrition for your brain because there is not a lot of information available about that. A nutrition plan should be individualized for you by you. Only you know your particular needs and what will help you stick with your plan.

One of the first things to consider is that a good nutrition plan should be enjoyable and easy to maintain. Eating is an important part of life that is associated with pleasure. When we think of a diet as something that restricts us and deprives us, we are not likely to keep doing it. As we talk about what is good for you in recovery, you need to think about not only how your nutrition can support recovery but also how enjoyable it will be.

Why Is Nutrition So Important in Recovery?

Food is the fuel the brain uses to function. And when your brain is not functioning properly you will feel unwell, unhappy, or anxious. Your stress levels will rise and stimulus augmentation will be heightened. You will not be able to think clearly and you will probably not sleep well. You will begin craving something—anything—to fill up the emptiness. If you want to feel good and enjoy life, you need to adequately feed your brain.

Proper nutrition is essential for a happy and healthy brain. We need protein, carbohydrates, and fat to provide energy, maintain the body, and feed the brain. Vitamins enable the body to properly utilize the protein, carbohydrates, and fat. Minerals (in addition to building bones and teeth, carrying oxygen to body cells, and maintaining muscle) help vitamins work efficiently. Water performs many functions and is essential to the survival of all cells. Fiber performs a useful role in digestion and provides a feeling of satisfaction.

Foods and Mood

In considering how food builds and maintains the body, let's not forget its very vital role in altering and maintaining mood. Depending on what amino acids they contain, some foods increase mental alertness, concentration, and energy while others are natural tranquilizers that calm feelings of anxiety and stress. But foods that calm you can also cause you to feel drowsy and mentally sluggish. What you eat and when you eat it can play an important part in your mood. Let's face it: *We self-regulate our mood continually with food.* Most of the time, we really don't know what we are doing and go for the quick fix rather than long-term well-being. To maintain sobriety and feel good it is imperative that you be familiar with the various types of foods and the nutrition they supply.

Foods for Alertness

As you already know, the neurotransmitter tyrosine is synthesized into dopamine and norepinephrine, increasing energy and alertness. Foods highest in tyrosine are foods derived from animal protein: chicken, turkey, pork, beef, dairy, and eggs. Moderate amounts of tyrosine are found in plant foods such as beans, corn, spinach, oatmeal, nuts, and seeds.

Foods for Relaxation

The neurotransmitter tryptophan, synthesized to serotonin, promotes relaxation and sleep. Foods high in tryptophan include turkey, green leafy vegetables, dairy products, bananas, pineapple, avocado, lentils, sesame seeds, and pumpkin. There are not many foods that contain tryptophan and those that do may not contain amounts sufficient to make it past the blood-brain barrier if they are competing with other amino acids, especially tyrosine. However, carbohydrates help carry the tryptophan to the brain. If you eat a carbohydrate-rich meal early in the day it can cause drowsiness. It is better to eat tryptophan-rich foods and carbohydrates in the evening when you want to relax and prepare for sleep rather than for breakfast when you want to become alert and energized. A good bedtime snack is milk and toast. The bread will help the tryptophan in the milk reach your brain and help you sleep.

Protein, Protein, Protein

A very important thing to know about a diet for recovery is that *protein contains all of the essential amino acids*. Therefore, a high-protein diet will give your brain more of the amino acids essential for its health. Think protein, protein, protein. Complete protein foods include meat, poultry, fish, eggs, and dairy products.

Protein not only feeds your brain and gives you energy, it also provides the body with the material it needs to replace worn tissue, fight infection, manufacture hormones and enzymes, and digest food. The body is damaged by heavy use of alcohol and other drugs and needs protein for rebuilding. The body stores very little protein, so you should eat it at least three times a day. And for enough energy—and your brain's sake—we recommend three meals and three snacks daily. You will probably feel best if your diet contains around 30 percent protein. And remember that most protein foods are rich in tyrosine.

High-Protein Cautions

Keep in mind that high-protein diets do require some cautions. Before you go on a high-protein diet, get a physical examination to make sure your kidneys are healthy and functioning well. Do not go on a high-protein diet if you have any kind of kidney problem. The kidneys are forced to work harder when they have to process protein as opposed to carbohydrates.

Diets that contain significant amounts of red meat may increase the risk of cancer. So, here are some words of advice about eating red meat.

- Cook meat slowly with lower heat. Try baked or crock pot meals such as stews. High heat causes carcinogens to form.
- Broil rather than grill.
- Avoid nitrite-cured meats. Most cured cold cuts and meats such as hot dogs, bacon, and ham contain nitrites that can spur formation of carcinogenic nitrosamines.

Red meat is usually high in fat—the bad saturated fat. A diet high in harmful fat poses many risks including that of heart disease. A high-protein diet that is high in harmful fat is not a good idea regardless of the benefit to your brain chemistry.

Low-Fat Protein Foods

But there are other good sources of animal protein that are low in fat or that contain good fat. Poultry and fish are, of course, the well-known ones. Fish is one of the most important ingredients in your diet which we will discuss in more detail later. But most of us get tired of a steady diet of chicken and fish. Try some alternatives.

Buffalo meat is red meat that is lower in fat than chicken but very tasty. If you have a hard time finding buffalo meat, get a group together and ask your grocer to stock it. Or you can order it yourself by calling Shepherd Farms at 660-261-4567. (Tell Dan and Janet that we told you to call.) We personally vouch for the quality of this source. We know that Shepherd Farms is careful about how their animals are fed and slaughtered, and the meat will come directly from them. We have been buying buffalo from them for about ten years.

Wild game also is usually low in fat and high in amino acids, so give it a try. Here's a great recipe for chili made with buffalo meat that you may want to try.

Dave's Buffalo Chili

2 lbs. ground buffalo
1 30-1/2 oz. can chili beans
1 28-oz. can diced tomatoes
1 pkg. Williams' Chili Seasoning*
1 Tbsp. B-V concentrate
1 large onion
1 can V-8 juice

Brown ground buffalo in skillet. Place in crock pot with other ingredients. Slow cook for 6-8 hours.

*no salt, msg, or preservatives added

Other sources of low-fat or good-fat protein high in tyrosine are eggs, yogurt, feta cheese, and cottage cheese. Be creative and find ways to enjoy low-fat, high-tyrosine foods to increase your energy and your ability to concentrate.

Fats

Don't be afraid of fat. Fat provides the most concentrated source of energy, supplies essential fatty acids, and enables the body to absorb certain vitamins. Like carbohydrates, there are good fats and bad fats. Without enough of the right types of fats, the brain is deprived of critical nutrients and the possibility of depression and other mental disorders increases. The goal is not to lower your fat consumption but to lower your consumption of unhealthy fats.

Our bodies need fat, and if we don't consume enough fat to give the body the energy it needs, we will crave simple carbs for fuel. An excellent way to relieve cravings for carbohydrates is to eat plenty of good fat. It is essential to your health and important to your recovery to learn which fats are good and which are bad for you.

Fats can be saturated, monounsaturated, or polyunsaturated. These designations refer to the types of bonds that hold their carbon atom chains together. Trans-fatty acids, another type of fat, are created through hydrogenation.

Saturated fatty acids are primarily found in red meat and dairy products. You should eat most saturated fatty acids sparingly because the liver manufactures cholesterol, especially LDLs (the bad cholesterol) from them. You do not, however, want to eliminate them entirely from your diet, because they constitute at least 50 percent of cell membranes, giving them firmness and integrity. Saturated fatty acids play a vital role in maintaining healthy bones.[1] They lower Lp(a), a substance in the blood associated with heart disease.[2] Saturated fatty acids are needed by the body to utilize essential fatty acids.[3] The fat around the heart muscle is mostly saturated fat, and the heart draws on this reserve of fat in times of stress.[4]

Eggs are a good source of saturated fat. Another good source is virgin coconut oil, which we will discuss shortly.

Monounsaturated fat is good fat. Olive oil and canola oil contain high amounts of monounsaturated fatty acids, 80 and 70 percent, respectively. The high consumption of olive oil in Mediterranean countries is considered to be one of the reasons why these countries have lower levels of heart disease.

Monounsaturated fat is believed to lower cholesterol and may assist in reducing heart disease. It provides essential fatty acids for healthy skin and the development of cells. Monounsaturated fat is also believed to offer protection against certain cancers, such as breast cancer and colon cancer.

Monounsaturated fats are typically high in vitamin E, an antioxidant vitamin that is usually in short supply in many Western diets. Cold-pressed extra-virgin olive oil, if not overheated, provides a range of phytochemicals and phenols that help to boost immunity and maintain good health. In addition to olive oil and canola oil, avocados, flaxseed, and most nuts also have high amounts of monounsaturated fat.

Polyunsaturated fatty acids have two or more double bonds. Oils that contain a high percentage of polyunsaturated fatty acids come from the following: corn, safflower, sunflower, peanut, cottonseed, soybean, fish, walnut, and flaxseed. Flaxseed oil and fish oil are the most highly unsaturated of all oils.

Fatty acids are the building blocks of fat. Essential fatty acids are necessary for human growth and cannot be manufactured in the body so we must get them from our diet. There are two families of essential fatty acids: omega-6 fatty acids and omega-3 fatty acids.

Most Americans consume adequate amounts of omega-6 fatty acids. The ratio of omega-6 to omega-3 fatty acids in your diet should be about 4:1. The typical Western diet contains approximately fourteen to twenty times more omega-6 fatty acids than omega-3s. Omega-6 fatty acids are most abundant in refined vegetable oils and red meat. Omega-3 fatty acids are found in foods such as fish, flaxseed oil, olive oil, and krill oil.

Fish Oil

Omega-3 fatty acids are found primarily in oily fish, such as salmon, sardines, halibut, and mackerel. Fish oil deficiency has been closely linked to addiction and co-existing conditions, such as depression, anxiety, ADHD, cognitive impairment, and sleep disorders. You can consume an adequate amount of omega-3 fatty acids by eating three servings of fish a week. Of course, the benefits of fish will be counteracted if you fry fish in harmful

Omega-3 Oil Increases Size or Volume of Brain Structures Associated with Mood

People who have lower blood levels of omega-3 fatty acids are more likely to have a negative outlook and be more impulsive. Conversely, people with higher blood levels of omega-3 fatty acids were found to be more agreeable and less likely to report mild or moderate symptoms of depression.

Human participants who had high levels of long-chain omega-3 fatty acid intake had higher volumes of gray matter in areas of the brain associated with emotional arousal and regulation. These are the same areas where gray matter is reduced in people who have mood disorders such as major depressive disorder.

Sarah M. Conklin[5]

fat or even good fat that changes its form when heated. Broil or bake your fish or fry it in palm oil or coconut oil (which will be discussed below). If you don't eat fish three times a week, be sure to take fish oil supplements.

Krill Oil

In a perfect world, you would be able to get all the omega-3s you need by eating fish. But perhaps you do not like fish. Or perhaps you are rightfully concerned about studies that show that eating fish can potentially expose you to a high degree of contamination with industrial pollutants and toxins, such as mercury, PCBs, heavy metals, and radioactive poisons.

Fortunately, you can get the same benefits from krill oil. Krill are shrimp-like marine invertebrates. Krill oil is very stable because it contains potent antioxidants that protect the oil. Fish oil is very perishable. It has been claimed that krill oil is perhaps one of the best brain-building foods available. Krill oil improves concentration, memory, learning, and mood. In addition to being a good brain food, krill oil is good for your heart, joints, cell membranes, liver, immune system, and skin.

Extra-Virgin Olive Oil

The greatest exponent of monounsaturated fat is olive oil. Olive oil is a natural juice, the only vegetable oil that can be consumed as it comes from the fruit. The beneficial health effects of olive oil are due to both its high content of monounsaturated fatty acids and its high content of antioxidants.

Olive oil is very well tolerated by the stomach. In fact, olive oil's protective function has a beneficial effect on ulcers and gastritis.

Generally, olive oil is extracted by pressing or crushing olives. Olive oil comes in different varieties, depending on the amount of processing involved. Varieties include:

- Extra virgin: considered the best, least processed, comprising the oil from the first pressing of the olives.
- Virgin: from the second pressing.
- Pure: undergoes some processing, such as filtering and refining.
- Light: undergoes considerable processing and only retains a very mild olive flavor.

When buying olive oil, look for a high-quality extra-virgin oil. The less the olive oil is handled, the closer to its natural state, the better the oil. Keep olive oil in a cool and dark place, tightly sealed. Oxygen promotes rancidity. Do not buy into the hype that canola (rapeseed) oil is superior to olive oil due to its concentration of monounsaturated fatty acids. Olive oil is far superior and has been around for thousands of years. If the taste of olive oil is a problem, or if you are frying or sautéing food, then you should consider coconut oil.

Virgin Coconut Oil[6]

We have very good news about coconut oil. It is good for you. That is, virgin coconut oil—or extra-virgin coconut oil. (Virgin and extra-virgin coconut oil are the same thing. Some manufacturers or retailers refer to virgin coconut oil as extra virgin. There is no difference in processing as there is with virgin and extra-virgin olive oil.) There is a difference, however, between virgin coconut oil and RBD coconut oil. RBD stands for refined, bleached, and deodorized. It is made from copra, the dried meat of the coconut. Virgin coconut oil, which is made from fresh coconut meat, is visibly clear and retains the scent and taste of coconuts.

Many nutritionally misinformed people consider use of coconut oil unwise due its nearly exclusive content of saturated fat. To understand why this is not true it is necessary to understand the chemical structure or the length of fatty acid chains.

Coconut oil is comprised of medium-chain fatty acids (MCFAs). Coconut oil is nature's richest source of these healthy fatty acids. Most vegetable or seed oils are composed of long-chain fatty acids (LCFAs). LCFAs are difficult for the body to break down, and they put more strain on the pancreas, the liver, and the digestive system. LCFAs are predominantly stored in the body as fat.

The MCFAs in coconut oil are healthier than LCFAs because they are smaller, so they permeate cell membranes easily. They are easily digested and are sent directly to your liver where they are immediately converted into energy rather than being stored as fat. Due to its stability and resistance to oxidation and free-radical formation, you can store coconut oil at room temperature for two years or more and it will not become rancid. However, don't store it in direct sunlight.

In the 1930s, Dr. Weston Price, a dentist, traveled throughout the South Pacific examining traditional diets and their effect on dental and overall health. He found that those who ate diets high in coconut products were healthy and trim, despite the high fat concentration in their diet.

Similarly, in 1981, researchers studied populations on two Polynesian atolls. Coconut was the chief source of caloric energy in both groups. The results, published in the *American Journal of Clinical Nutrition*, demonstrated that both populations exhibited positive vascular health. There was no evidence that the high saturated fat intake had a harmful effect in these populations.

Extra-virgin olive oil is healthier than coconut oil if it is not heated. It is an omega-3 fat and works great as a salad dressing. However, it is not the best oil to cook with. Due to its chemical structure, cooking makes it susceptible to oxidative damage. And polyunsaturated fats—which include common vegetable oils such as corn, soy, safflower, sunflower, and canola—are the worst oils to use in cooking. This is because their double bonds are highly susceptible to heat damage. Frying destroys the antioxidants in these oils and oxidizes the oils, which causes far more damage than trans fats.

Coconut oil is the only oil that is stable enough to resist heat-induced damage, so you can use coconut oil instead of butter, olive oil, vegetable oil, or any other type of oil called for in recipes. Coconut oil is very stable even at high temperatures. However, it is best not to heat it beyond its smoke point as this will deteriorate the oil and turn it yellow. (If coconut oil has turned dark yellow it should be discarded.) The smoke point of coconut oil can be increased by combining it with virgin palm oil. Both of these oils have a much higher smoke point and are suitable for high heat, even for deep frying.

You have probably heard that breast milk is packed with nutrients and disease-fighting ingredients that help keep babies healthy. Coconut oil contains one of the same compounds (lauric acid) that helps strengthen the immune system. Lauric acid is the predominant type of MCFA in coconut oil. In fact, a volume of research has been done establishing the ability of lauric acid to enhance immunity. Outside of mother's milk, coconut oil is nature's most plentiful source of lauric acid.

The numerous health benefits of coconut oil are finally reaching the mainstream. Benefits include promoting heart health, promoting proper weight maintenance, supporting the immune system, improving metabolism, providing an immediate energy source, keeping skin healthy, and supporting healthy thyroid function. To get full health benefits of coconut oil, try to consume three to four tablespoons per day.

Just a word or two of caution: Be sure to purchase virgin coconut oil that has not been refined, has no chemicals added, has no hydrogenation, and is made without heat processing. And don't pay any attention to some ads that claim that their coconut oil is better because it is more raw and therefore contains more enzymes. If coconut oil contained enzymes it would quickly deteriorate and would not have some of the benefits we have been telling you about. Also we want to be sure you don't think that you are getting omega-3 fatty acids in coconut oil. There are none. You still need to get those from fish, fish oil, and other foods high in omega-3.

In our home, coconut oil is a mainstay. It is the only oil we use, (except for olive oil on salads). It enables us to enjoy fried food, which we considered off limits before we discovered the health benefits of coconut oil. And remember what we said earlier: You are more apt to stick with healthy eating if you enjoy it. With coconut oil you can fry, stir-fry, or sauté. You can make your own mayonnaise. And for a dose of lauric acid, you can put some into a smoothie or other healthy snack. So enjoy. No cholesterol. No trans-fats. No guilt. No downside.

Avoid Trans-Fatty Acids

Trans-fatty acids behave in many ways like saturated fat, including raising your LDL (bad) cholesterol. They are formed through a process of heating vegetable oil into solids like margarine and shortening (hydrogenating). They are often added to processed foods, allowing them to be shipped in warm, humid weather and left on grocery stores' shelves for months. Look for the words *hydrogenated* or *partially hydrogenated* in the list of ingredients to see if trans-fat is included. Trans-fatty acids push both blood cholesterol levels (LDL and HDL) in the wrong direction. They also interfere with essential fatty acid metabolism.

Foods high in trans-fatty acids include: biscuit mixes and dough, cakes and cake mixes, cinnamon rolls, cookies and cookie mixes, corn chips, crackers, doughnuts, granola, frozen desserts (not ice cream), muffin mixes, pastries in general, pie crusts and pie crust mixes, popcorn (flavored), potato chips, shortening, tortillas, and tortilla chips. The good news is that more of these foods are now being produced without trans-fatty acids. Be sure to read the labels so you'll know what you are buying.

Carbohydrates

Carbohydrates are a major energy source and help us use other nutrients. Carbohydrates also help produce serotonin. The low-carb craze may have you thinking that carbs are bad for you. Like fat, however, there are good carbs and bad carbs. And you need the good carbs—for energy and for serotonin production.

When the body digests food, it converts carbohydrates to a type of sugar called glucose. As the level of glucose rises in the bloodstream, the pancreas releases insulin which helps move the glucose into the body's many cells. Once glucose enters the cells it is either burned for energy or converted to and stored as fat.

There are two types of carbohydrates: simple and complex. The big difference is in how quickly the body processes them into glucose. Simple carbs are processed quickly, while complex carbs are processed more slowly. The rate at which foods are processed into glucose is sometimes referred to as the glycemic load. Simple carbs are primarily sweets and white flour foods, and complex carbs are whole grains, legumes, and some vegetables and nuts.

The problem with simple carbs is that they give you a surge of energy that is soon followed by a letdown. This occurs because the pancreas releases insulin to compensate for the rush of sugar. The body then releases adrenaline to remove the insulin, which in turn produces that letdown feeling, which triggers a desire for more sweets to raise your blood sugar level for another surge of energy. If your blood sugar is low, you may feel moody, fatigued, confused, anxious, and irritable. All your chronic abstinence symptoms are intensified. Simple carbohydrates, then, contribute to mood swings, low energy, and cravings.

Complex carbohydrates are also made up of sugars, but the sugar molecules are strung together to form longer, more complex chains, so they're absorbed more gradually into the bloodstream. As a result, your brain does not get the sudden surge of sugar that it gets from simple carbs. Complex carbohydrates provide energy without the surge and without the letdown. They also give you a wider array of vitamins and minerals that your body cannot get from a strict high-protein diet. A complex carbohydrate snack in the evening with some milk will provide tryptophan to increase serotonin to help you relax and sleep.

The Story of the Potato

The potato is a paradoxical food. For a while, we were told that potatoes were high in starch (sugar) and should be eaten sparingly. At one time, First Lady Rosalynn Carter announced that her family was going to start eating better and cut out potatoes. But the potato industry responded by telling us it is not the potato, but what we put on it that is bad, and that potatoes are high in many of the vitamins and minerals we need. Good for us without the bad toppings. So some of us learned to enjoy our potatoes plain, leaving off the butter and sour cream. Recently, we have been hit with some bad news again. It is the potato. Researchers are telling us that eating a baked potato is the same as eating a half cup of sugar. Oh, wow! But they aren't telling us the whole story. That is true only if you eat it plain, on an empty stomach, with nothing on it or with it. Butter or sour cream slows the absorption process so it goes into the blood stream more slowly. If you substitute a good fat for butter or use low-fat sour cream, you can get the many nutrients in potatoes without spiking your blood sugar.

While we've presented a lot of information about nutrition, remember that the most important thing is to be moderate and sensible. Try to replace bad fats with good fats, bad carbs with good carbs. If you eat simple carbs once in a while, try to eat them with high fiber or good-fat foods. (Fiber and fat slow the rate at which carbohydrates are absorbed into the bloodstream.) And eat them late in the day when you want to relax rather than when you want to be alert.

In addition to selecting whole grains instead of processed grains and restricting white foods, here are some other ways you can get the serotonin and nutritional benefits of carbohydrates while lowering your glycemic load:

- Eat more legumes (dried beans, lentils and nuts).
- Eat more high-fiber fruits and vegetables.
- Add vinegar or lemon juice to carbs; the acid lowers the glycemic load as much as 30 percent. Eat a green salad with acidic dressing along with carbohydrate foods.
- Choose old-fashioned or steel-ground oatmeal over highly processed cereals.
- Eat brown rice and basmati rice, as well as wild rice (not actually rice but high in fiber, has a low glycemic load, and tastes very good).
- Eat a bit of protein or good fat along with carbohydrates.
- Exercise daily.

Sugar and Other Sweeteners

We have been pointing out that simple carbohydrates are not the best choice for your diet. However, most people enjoy something sweet at least occasionally. If you eat sugar once in a while, do it in moderation. Avoid concentrated sweets such as sugared soft drinks, pies, cake icing, and candy. You can also eat things that are sweetened with substances other than processed sugar. But there are some things you need to consider when you do.

Honey and molasses are simple carbohydrates and cause the same reaction in your brain as refined sugar. Honey does have trace amounts of vitamins not found in processed sugar and it is also an antioxidant. But it is still a simple carb and will have the same effect on your blood sugar and mood as other simple carbs. If the choice is between sugar and honey, choose honey. But it is best to avoid both and get your vitamins and antioxidants in other ways.

Many people replace sugar with artificial sweeteners, but there is some controversy as to whether or not some artificial sweeteners are safe. Most are better for you than sugar and some of the reports and messages about them have been promoted by the sugar industry. Don't believe everything you hear, but it doesn't hurt to be cautious.

Processed fructose is a good choice if you aren't worried about the calories. It does not require insulin to make it available for energy in the body so it does not affect blood sugar levels. Fructose adds the same number of calories as sugar, however, so you don't hear much about it as most people want to avoid excess calories. (Don't take this to mean that all fruit is sweetened with fructose and therefore doesn't affect blood sugar. Different fruits have different sugars. Grapes are primarily sucrose.)

Complementary Protein

Although it is important to consume the full range of amino acids, it is not necessary to get them all from meat, fish, poultry, and other complete protein foods. In fact, because of their high fat content—as well as the use of antibiotics and other chemicals in the raising of poultry and cattle—most of those foods should be eaten in moderation only. Complete protein contains all the essential amino acids. Complex carbohydrates (incomplete protein) contain some of them. You can combine partial protein foods to make complete protein. These are grains, legumes, and some leafy green vegetables. Brown rice and beans each lacks one or more of the necessary amino acids for complete protein. But when you combine the two, or when you combine either one with any number of other complex carbohydrate foods, you form a complete protein that is a high-quality substitute for meat. To make a complete protein, combine beans with brown rice, corn, nuts, seeds, or wheat.

As a matter of fact, combinations of legumes (such as beans, peanuts, peas) with almost any grains, nuts, or seeds will make a complete protein. In addition, cornmeal fortified with the amino acid L-lysine makes a complete protein. A meal of beans and corn bread provides complete protein without meat.

Another good way of adding protein to meals is to add nuts and seeds to salads and vegetable casseroles. Add protein-rich snacks as often as possible. Eat whole-grain bread with nut butters or a handful of nuts and seeds.

Remember, plant protein does not provide as much tyrosine as animal sources. If you choose to get your protein by reducing meat intake and consuming more combined carbohydrates, you may want to also add a little cottage cheese, skim milk, or eggs if you need the tyrosine. Of course, another option is to supplement with tyrosine capsules.

Vitamins and Minerals

Vitamins enable the body to use the protein, carbohydrates, and fat for fuel and maintenance. We need a variety of foods, particularly fruits and vegetables, to get all the essential vitamins. You should eat five to eight servings of fruits and vegetables a day. Vitamin B12 (without which we develop pernicious anemia) is available only in animal foods. If you are a vegetarian, make sure you take a vitamin B12 supplement.

Minerals are necessary for building healthy bones and teeth, for carrying oxygen to body cells, and for maintaining muscle tone. They also help vitamins work efficiently. Calcium, necessary for building and maintaining bones and teeth, is found primarily in dairy products. Because dairy foods are characteristically high in fat, you should take special care to get adequate calcium if you reduce your fat intake. You can eat low-fat dairy products such as yogurt and low-fat cheeses, or get calcium from green leafy vegetables such as broccoli and collard greens.

Fiber

Fiber has no nutritive value, but it performs a useful role in digestion. Fiber contributes to good health and provides a feeling of satisfaction when we eat. It increases the feeling of satiation and reduces hunger and craving. High-fiber foods require more chewing, which helps us to eat more slowly, and slow eaters usually feel more satisfied. High-fiber foods include whole grains, fruits and vegetables, and seeds.

When to Eat

Very simply, you need to eat tyrosine-rich foods when you want to be alert and tryptophan-rich foods when you want to relax. To avoid hunger, eat several times during the day. How often you eat can vary, but it is important not to get hungry. We should eat smaller amounts more often to avoid getting hungry and eating the wrong foods. In recovery one of the major things we are trying to accomplish is to avoid cravings. Hunger creates cravings. And when you are really hungry, you will eat whatever is fastest, not what is best for you.

A nutritious breakfast provides the initial energy we need; it sets us up to function well throughout the day. Sara used to go all day without eating, thinking she was cutting calories. But by dinner time she would grab the fastest and easiest foods she could find, because she was too hungry to take time to cook. Usually the most convenient foods are not the most nutritious or the most satisfying. Once she started eating, she found it difficult to stop. She ended up eating more than if she had eaten breakfast and lunch. Now that her self-care plan includes eating regular meals, she has more energy all day long. She now realizes she was depriving her body of the fuel it needed for her busy life.

Avoiding Trigger Foods

Trigger foods are those that, when eaten, cause you to want to eat more—and more. Sweets are the most common trigger food. Complex carbohydrates are less likely to trigger cravings, and are much easier to eat in reasonable amounts. Balance, balance, balance is the watchword. Carbohydrate binges are less likely to occur if you balance your carbs with high protein rather than trying to eliminate them completely.

If you attend a meeting of Alcoholics Anonymous you will usually find lots of coffee, lots of cigarette smoke, and oftentimes a platter of donuts. It has been found that when alcoholics stop drinking or other drug addicts give up their drug of choice, they increase their intake of sugar, caffeine, and nicotine. Why? Because they need something to satisfy the craving created by removing the drug upon which they were dependent.

While this is sometimes encouraged or at least justified with the statement that eating sweets is better than drinking, in the long run, it is not a good alternative. Yes, for an alcoholic, eating sweets is better than drinking. But the fact is, it does not reduce craving and may make it more difficult to stay sober. The cravings that continues to plague the abstinent addict are an indication that the underlying problem has not been addressed. The brain is still crying out for something it is not getting.

How does the brain get what it needs to eliminate craving and provide a sense of well-being? Remember, craving is a neurotransmitter problem; neurotransmitters are made from amino acids. So what is the brain crying out for? Right—proper nutrition.

Sugar and caffeine do not work to relieve cravings. It only seems like it at the moment. Like other drugs, they provide temporary relief. But the relief is quickly replaced by intensified craving. So these new substances create the same cycle of relief and craving that the drug of choice previously provided. And alcoholics or heroin addicts soon find themselves addicted to the substitute. What works is feeding the brain what it needs for neurotransmitter replacement.

There is a wide variety of opinion about the extent to which we should avoid trigger foods. Some people say trigger foods are like alcohol for an alcoholic and should be eliminated entirely, but for most people that is unrealistic. For some of us, the sense of deprivation that comes from identifying forbidden foods— foods we can never eat—creates stronger cravings than eating the foods in moderation.

There is no simple answer to this. And there certainly is not one that applies to everyone. But it is important to recognize that nutrition is an important part of recovery and that certain foods can trigger cravings for foods that do not feed our brains. But if you believe that by permanently depriving yourself of certain foods you risk bingeing on them to relieve the pain of feeling deprived, include them in your nutrition plan in a controlled way. Some people allow a treat periodically as part of their nutrition plan to relieve feelings of unrelenting deprivation. To eat the treat in moderation, follow a control plan for managing the craving that is triggered.

Sue occasionally gets a small ice cream cone, away from home, and then takes a walk in the park. She takes a small bag of nuts (high in protein) with her to offset the sugar. When the ice cream is gone, more is not readily available, and the exercise helps to relieve the craving. For her, this is much better than eating a bowl of ice cream at home. Ice cream in the freezer continues to call to her until she goes and gets more—and more and more.

When you eat a high-protein diet you will be surprised to find that cravings are greatly reduced, even for carbohydrates. If your tendency is to grab a cookie when you are uncomfortable and find yourself bingeing on sweets, try eating some protein or complex carbohydrates instead of the cookies. You will feel more satisfied and less tempted to go for the ice cream. You will have more energy and feel less anxious. Your brain is getting what it needs to produce the feel-good neurotransmitters that need to be replenished.

Caffeine

Caffeine stimulates the release of neurotransmitters that make you feel energized. In moderation caffeine will not hurt you. But five or six cups of coffee or bottles of cola a day can cause high anxiety. And you can become addicted to caffeine. If you find yourself drinking more than two or three cups of coffee a day or gradually increasing the amount you drink, you should cut back or stop completely. The key word is definitely moderation.

But for those of you who are tea drinkers, there is good news—it's good for you. A new study[3] suggests that drinking green or black tea slows the time it takes for LDL (bad cholesterol) to become oxidized, a process that is thought to be important in the formation of fatty plaques in coronary arteries. Tea contains flavonoids. Flavonoids are a group of polyphenolic antioxidants that are contained in vegetables, fruit, and beverages such as tea or wine. Most tea studies conducted in China or Japan focus on green tea, the type of tea most often consumed in those countries. However, in the new study the participants drank black tea, which is most often consumed in Western nations. Both teas are derived from the same plant but are the results of different processing methods. Green tea and black tea appear to be reasonably equivalent in terms of antioxidant properties.

12 Steps for Nutritious Eating

1. Eat nutrient-dense foods: Limit intake of simple carbohydrates, avoid empty-calorie junk foods.
2. Learn to read labels: Avoid overly processed foods with artificial ingredients and preservatives.
3. Eat 5–8 servings of fresh fruits and vegetables daily.
4. Get plenty of omega-3 fatty acids: Eat 2–3 servings of oily fish weekly and consume nuts and seeds daily.
5. Consume a balance of good fats; avoid bad fats. Use only coconut oil for cooking.
6. Eat three small meals and three snacks daily, beginning each day with a nutritious, balanced breakfast.
7. Snack between meals on nuts, seeds, fresh fruits (especially berries), and dark chocolate.
8. Eat slowly and chew thoroughly.
9. Supplement daily with amino acids, vitamins, and minerals.
10. Drink purified water (reverse osmosis preferred).
11. Avoid fruit juices: Chew your foods; don't drink them.
12. Avoid soft drinks and minimize coffee consumption; drink green tea or black tea instead.

Thanks to Bridging the Gaps for contributing to this list.

Weight

Many chemically addicted people are either overweight or underweight due to poor eating habits. Proper eating habits will probably correct an underweight problem fairly rapidly. A problem with obesity is not usually as easily corrected. A person can be overweight and still suffer from malnutrition. A weight reduction program should be undertaken carefully, with the help and advice of a physician.

Immediate weight loss in early sobriety may not be wise because of the stress related to dieting. This, along with the stress of adjusting to sobriety and a new lifestyle, may be more than you are ready to cope with. Talk to your doctor. It may be wise to establish and practice a good nutritional program along with making the other lifestyle adjustments necessary for recovery before thinking of losing weight.

If you decide to lose weight, do so sensibly. Beware of rapid weight-loss diets. They can be harmful to your health and very stressful. Be satisfied with gradual loss. Continue to eat a balanced diet and avoid hunger. Increase your exercise as well as decreasing calories. It is the combination that makes for the most successful weight-loss plan. A focus on good health rather than attaining an unrealistic weight goal usually achieves the best results.

A Modified Mediterranean Diet

We understand that figuring out how to eat nutritiously can be complicated and inconvenient sometimes, so we are going to recommend an eating plan for you that can make your life simpler while you enjoy healthy eating. The closest diet to what we have been recommending is the Mediterranean Diet. You can modify it according to your own preferences and according to some of the suggestions we have already made.

The Mediterranean Diet is a way of eating that cultures throughout the Mediterranean have practiced for centuries. Scientific studies have associated this type of diet with longer lives and less chronic diseases in countries throughout the Mediterranean. This diet is characterized by the following:

• High intake of vegetables, fruits, legumes, nuts, and seeds; whole-grain cereals and pastas; healthy monounsaturated fats like olive oil.
• Moderate-to-high intake of wild-caught fish
• Moderate intake of eggs and poultry; low fat dairy products
• Low intake of red meat and saturated fatty acids from meats and dairy.

Good nutrition feeds the brain. A well-functioning brain is the key to long-term sobriety. While this is sometimes mentioned in conventional treatment and occasionally in AA, it is seldom emphasized. The role of nutrition cannot be overstated. Addiction is a disease of the brain. Recovery requires feeding the brain.

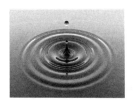

CHAPTER 7

Acupuncture, Auriculotherapy, and Cranial Electrical Stimulation

IN THE LAST FEW YEARS, acupuncture and auricular therapy have been used increasingly to treat substance abuse disorders. Though more research is needed, numerous studies have validated the use of these therapies. Since scientific research shows that addiction, withdrawal, and chronic abstinence symptoms are related to chemicals in the nervous system and to stress regulating hormones in the body, it is reasonable that all remedies that affect these systems be explored when seeking therapy that works in the treatment of addiction.

Acupuncture[1]

Acupuncture dates back thousands of years, yet in the United States it has only recently begun to be recognized as a valid form of treatment for a variety of health conditions. While there is still skepticism among medical practitioners, there is strong evidence that it works, especially in the alleviation of pain. It has been used successfully as anesthesia for animals—and placebos don't work with animals.

Traditionally, acupuncture healers seek to restore the balance of two complementary energy forces (yin and yang) that travel through the body by way of channels called meridians. These energy forces crisscross the arms, legs, trunk, and head and course deep within the tissues. These energy forces must be in balance for our vital life functions—including physical, emotional, mental, and spiritual states—to operate correctly. The meridians surface at various locations—called acupuncture points—on the body, each of which is associated with one or more specific organs. The idea is that the organs can be influenced by stimulating an appropriate acupuncture point.

Acupuncture involves stimulation of these points on the skin with ultra fine needles that are manipulated manually, and sometimes electrically. It is said that acupuncture moves energy. The ancient explanation for the effectiveness of acupuncture is that when conditions interfere with the energy flow through the meridians, toxins build up in the body and block body systems from functioning optimally. Stimulating acupuncture points releases the energy flow, and balance is restored.

Western scientists suggest a different or additional explanation for the effectiveness of acupuncture: mobilization of opioids in the reward system of the brain. This theory is supported by the fact that experimental animals, when given naloxone (a chemical that blocks opioids) do not respond to acupuncture. As we have stated previously, the opioid neurotransmitters reduce pain even more effectively than narcotics and without the side effects.

There is no tangible evidence of the existence of acupuncture meridians. They cannot be touched or dissected. However, under a microscope acupuncture points appear to have a greater concentration of nerve endings than other skin locations. And electric skin conductivity, which can be measured, is greater at these points.

Concerning the safety of acupuncture, there is always potential harm when a sharp instrument penetrates the body. However, professionals using sterilized needles will seldom do any harm. We advise that you make sure the needles used on you are disposable—the most sure method of preventing transmission of infections like HIV/AIDS and hepatitis. Most states require acupuncturists to pass a course on infection control and proper handling of equipment.

The FDA has approved the use of acupuncture needles as medical devices. Twenty-one states restrict the practice of acupuncture to licensed doctors; the other twenty-nine states and Washington, DC, permit non-physicians who complete a training course and pass a certifying exam to use acupuncture.

Specialists in pain management often use acupuncture. If you are a recovering addict and are abstaining from mood-altering substances, such as painkillers, acupuncture may be a good alternative for pain relief. People who suffer from back pain, bursitis, osteoarthritis, and headaches can benefit from acupuncture. In a study in California, eleven women plagued by recurring menstrual cramps were treated with acupuncture once a week. The same number of women received painkillers. After three months, ten of the women in the acupuncture group had significant relief. The others reported no change.[2]

Acu-detox (Ear Acupuncture)[3]

About 2,500 years ago, it was discovered that there are points in the ear that, when manipulated with needles, are effective in relieving the discomfort of withdrawal from opium. In more recent times Hsaing Lai Weng successfully applied electrical stimulation to needles inserted in the ear to relieve opiate withdrawal symptoms. Over several years Michael Smith, a physician at Lincoln Hospital in Bronx, New York, and his associates refined the detox protocol into five ear points that are manipulated with needles. To promote his protocol, Smith founded the National Acupuncture Detoxification Association. Currently his protocol is utilized in numerous settings including drug treatment programs, jails, prisons, and drug courts.

While acu-detox has been found to be very beneficial, keep in mind that it is limited to detoxification from opiate-type drugs such as heroin, methadone, barbiturates, and alcohol, but it has not been found to be helpful in detox from stimulants such as cocaine. And it is a detoxification tool, not a tool for ongoing recovery.

Ear acupuncture is an ancient discipline that has stood the test of time. Even though there is not strong scientific research to show how and why it works, there is plenty of anecdotal evidence to demonstrate its worth. When ear acupuncture is used in an inpatient detoxification setting, the severity of withdrawal is reduced and seizures can be controlled. It is usually done twice a day in a group setting for forty-five to ninety minutes.

Acupressure

Instead of using needles, some acupuncturists apply pressure to the designated points with their fingers or stick-like devices. Michael Smith at Lincoln Hospital uses beads or seeds taped to these points in the ear. He has found this helpful for babies born addicted to crack and with children diagnosed with ADHD.

Needle-less Auricular Therapy[4] (Auriculotherapy)

Although the term *auriculotherapy* is sometimes used to refer to any type of ear therapy, including ear acupuncture, we use it here to describe a needle-less procedure that utilizes four cranial nerves and three cervical ganglia within the ear, not acupuncture points. Auriculotherapy uses a microcurrent device to diagnose and treat those nerves that are a direct entry to the brain and spinal cord. Auriculotherapy is used to identify the location and measurement of an abnormal nerve point and then to treat that point with micro-amp current at a specific frequency depending on where the point is located.

Dr. Paul Nogier laid the groundwork of auriculotherapy in the 1950s. He discovered that auricular nerves form a microsystem. A microsystem is a small location in the body that represents the whole body. As with other microsystems—foot (reflexology), eye (iridology), scalp, or hand (Su Jok)—there are areas in the ear that correspond to specific systems of the body.

Nogier first used cautery to intervene at locations of the ear, then needles, and finally milli-amp current, which was the most successful. Later, other researchers upgraded to micro-amp current, which has worked the best and is almost imperceptible to the patient. These microcurrents were successful in relieving pain and caused no trauma to the patients.

Auriculotherapy practitioners use a hand-held device first to locate abnormal points of increased skin conductivity on the ear and then to treat those identified points. The nervous system is tonal, meaning that nerves function at a specific frequency, measured in hertz (Hz). Hertz is defined as cycles per second, or how many times something occurs within a second—its frequency. The auricular nerves function at 5 Hz, 10 Hz, or 20 Hz.

Auriculotherapy points manifest as points of increased skin conductivity only if there is a problem in the corresponding part of the body which the ear point represents. Once the points have been located, the microcurrent device is used to stimulate the nerve to decrease skin conductivity at that location. The less conductive, the healthier it is until finally when it is really healthy, it is not conductive at all. The point is gone, unlike acupuncture points that never disappear.

Auriculotherapy has its practical application in addiction treatment by causing the specific release of neurotransmitters that may be sluggish or in short supply in the addicted brain and spinal cord. The release of these neurotransmitters is stimulated by the application of microcurrent to the nerves in the ear that directly lead into the brain. The electrical current sends a message to increase the activity of the receptor site so that when the neurotransmitter arrives there and places itself in its receptor, the result will be magnified and enhanced. One reason this auriculotherapy is so successful in addiction treatment is that the nerves have direct entry to and from the brain—where the major portion of healing from addiction takes place.

Auriculotherapy is not paint-by-numbers. It is always specific to the needs of the individual receiving it. This is made possible because of the precise diagnostic capability of auriculotherapy's microcurrent and specific frequency.

When Paul Nogier first developed auriculotherapy—then termed auricular medicine—he was limited to electrical devices that were nine-volt powered, providing only a milli-amp current. So it was much less accurate in point location than today because of the inaccuracy of electronics of the age. Nogier didn't have integrated circuits, so there were all kinds of limitations. But auricular medicine has evolved into a highly accurate and objective procedure.

Unlike acupuncture points along meridians, points along the nerves are tangible; you can see them, you can dissect them, and you can measure them. They have a frequency because nerve tissue is tonal. Neurophysiology is very tangible.

The auriculotherapy approach to treatment is clearly defined. It has been found to be safe and effective and the microcurrent instrument has FDA approval. There are hundreds of diseases that auriculotherapy can diagnose and treat, but there are two areas for which it is most successful: pain management and addiction treatment. With pain management it is almost instantaneous; with addiction it is not instantaneous. For addiction recovery there is no quick fix. But this is where auriculotherapy is a plus. It is useful beyond the detoxification stage. Auriculotherapy is usually done initially in recovery after detox in a minimum of ten treatments in a row, five days a week for the first two weeks. We recommend twenty treatments within the first thirty days: five treatments a week.

Auriculotherapy goes beyond the limitations of acu-detox. It can be individualized for each person and for specific drugs and it is a faster procedure. When needles are used, as in acu-detox, they are inserted for forty-five to ninety minutes twice daily. However, needles are inert, do not have frequency or polarity capabilities. Better outcomes can be attained with auriculotherapy in fifteen minutes. With auriculotherapy the skin is not punctured, so treatment is safer. Dr. Jay Holder and Associates at Exodus Treatment Center in Miami have attained a 93 to 96 percent retention rate in residential treatment with the inclusion of auricular therapy.[5] To find an auriculotherapist near you, contact the American College of Addictionology and Compulsive Disorders at 800-490-7714 or 305-535-8803 or visit www.acacd.com.

Cranial Electrical Stimulation

Since the brain functions by utilizing electrical activity, it follows that mental functions can be influenced by altering the brain's electrical activity. Cranial electrical stimulation (CES) provides a gentle electrical current that stimulates the production of brain chemicals that increase a feeling of well-being.[6] CES stimulates the brain by means of two electrodes that are usually placed behind the ear or clipped to the upper portion of the ear lobe. Some clinicians apply the electrodes to the head and the wrist. A pocket-size control unit can be easily carried from place to place.

During CES, an electric current is focused on the hypothalamic region and promotes an increase in endorphins. The current results in an increase of the brain's levels of serotonin, norepinephrine, and dopamine, and a decrease in its level of cortisol. When CES is effective, users are in an alert, yet relaxed state, characterized by alpha brainwaves.

Electrotherapy has been used for at least 2,000 years, as shown by the clinical literature of the Roman physician Scribonius Largus, who wrote in the *Compositiones Medicae* in 46 AD that his patients should stand on a live black torpedo fish to relieve a variety of medical conditions, including gout and headaches. Modern research into low-intensity electrical stimulation of the brain was begun by Leduc and Rouxeau in France in 1902. In 1949, the Soviet Union expanded CES research to include the treatment of anxiety as well as sleep disorders.

Electrical devices have not caught on until recently. The use of prescription medications to the exclusion of other methods of treating the brain, along with the fear and stigma of using electrical devices on the brain (related to electroconvulsive therapy) has slowed the awareness and acceptance of the effectiveness and safety of electrical stimulation therapy. Public sentiment is beginning to change, however. There is increasing awareness that prescription drugs may not be the safest or most effective way to treat the brain. While CES is still a relatively unknown treatment option, it is gaining recognition for its effectiveness and safety.

Most users of CES report a decrease in anxiety in as little as two days and a noticeable reduction in anxiety within ten treatments. Some (but not all) users report a euphoric feeling. Most report that their thinking is clearer and that they feel more creative.

Studies indicate that low-voltage electrical brain stimulation is therapeutically beneficial in the treatment of conditions such as depression, substance-use disorder, withdrawal symptoms, and insomnia.[7] The FDA has cleared several CES units to be marketed for the treatment of anxiety, depression, and insomnia. There have been no major complications or negative effects associated with CES. A few users feel mild discomfort while using CES but suffer no long-term difficulties.

CES produces an increase in beta-endorphin levels and acetylcholine levels, which blocks anxiety and improves cognitive functioning. It can directly affect the stress levels connected with a reward deficiency in the brain by producing more relaxing, reward-enhancing brain chemistry.

CES has also been shown to significantly improve the P300 brainwave,[8] which has been associated with ADHD as it relates to both drug craving and attention span. Eric Braverman and his associates[9] have shown through brain mapping that many serious brain disorders have electrical rhythm disturbances. CES may normalize a variety of these rhythm disturbances.

(Thanks to Dr. Jay Holder for contributions to this chapter.)

CHAPTER 8

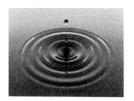

Brainwave Biofeedback
(Neurofeedback)

THE NERVOUS SYSTEM HAS TWO MAJOR COMPONENTS—voluntary and involuntary. The voluntary component is totally under your control. If you want to move your leg or arm, you simply decide to do it, and your brain does the rest. The brain sends a message, via the nerves down to the leg, and the leg moves. By contrast, the involuntary nervous system, which controls such body functions as heart rate, blood pressure, and skin temperature, operates out of conscious awareness and without conscious direction from you. However, you can learn to control or at least affect many of the involuntary mechanisms, including muscle tension, heart rate, blood supply to the skin, and even motions.

Biofeedback is a process by which you learn to recognize signals your body provides that tell you how it is functioning. When you weigh yourself or take your heart rate or check your blood pressure, you are receiving feedback from your body about your body.

Body temperature rises as you relax. Do you remember the mood rings that were popular a number of years ago? The ones that changed colors according to your mood? These rings provided a form of biofeedback, changing color as your body temperature changed. The same principle is operating with those stress dots that change color when you put your finger on them. As you relax, the dot or the ring changes color because your body temperature rises. Thermometers are another biofeedback tool. As you relax, your temperature will rise, and the thermometer becomes a biofeedback machine.

Mood rings, stress dots, and thermometers are real examples of how we can use biofeedback to have some control over involuntary body functions such as blood pressure, heart rate, and temperature. The more feedback you get, the better able you will be to control involuntary functions on demand and reduce pain, eliminate bad habits, and lower your blood pressure.

Neurofeedback

Neurofeedback (also called brainwave biofeedback and EEG biofeedback) is a technique by which you train the brain to regulate itself. Neurofeedback allows you to consciously change your mental states by helping you learn to increase or decrease the frequency of your brainwaves. It involves displaying a person's brainwaves on a computer screen and helping that person learn to control them.

Neurofeedback has a dual role. First, brainwaves displayed on a computer monitor can identify when the brain is not functioning well. With the same technology, it is possible control the brainwaves and enable the brain to function better. You can challenge the brain to function better just as you can challenge your muscles to function better with exercise.

Neurofeedback is noninvasive and quite simple. Electrodes

are attached to the scalp to monitor brainwaves. These electrodes are connected to a computer that supplies feedback as to what is occurring in the brain. Frequency is the rate at which electrical charges move through brain cells. The human brain is measured by four basic frequency ranges.

- *Delta*, the sleep state: very slow brainwaves; just 4 cycles (hertz [Hz]) per second.
- *Theta*, a deeply relaxed, daydreaming state, 4 to 8 Hz.
- *Alpha*, a relaxed but alert state, 8 to 13 Hz.
- *Beta*, the most rapid brainwaves, reflecting normal waking consciousness in a range from 12 to 35 Hz. (A relaxed but alert state of low beta is 12 to 15 Hz, mid-range beta is 15 to 19 Hz, an excited, hyper state of high beta can be as high as 35 Hz.)

It seems that problems occur when the brainwaves are either too slow or too fast. There is speculation that brainwave frequency may be a major component in a multitude of disorders. The goal of neurofeedback is to stabilize brainwave frequency.

Dale Walters, a friend and colleague who worked extensively with neurofeedback at the Menninger Clinic, in Topeka, Kansas, first introduced us to it for use with ADHD and addiction. It is now being used for closed head injury, post traumatic stress disorder, seizures, sleep disorders, depression, and Tourette's syndrome. And it can be used by anyone to promote relaxation and a sense of well-being and to enhance alertness.

Training Your Brain with Neurofeedback

Two things happen with neurofeedback training. First, you can learn self-regulation—that is, you can learn to alter your own brainwaves. You can learn how to speed up the frequency when you need to concentrate and to slow the frequency when you need to relax. Like other types of biofeedback, neurofeedback provides access to our internal processes and allows us to regulate them. The reward of successful self-regulation is the ability to relax if you are highly stressed or the ability to focus if you have trouble concentrating.

Second, with neurofeedback training, actual changes occur in the brain. People who use brain mapping or brain scans report that, as a result of neurofeedback, changes take place in the electrical activity of the brain that persist long term. Deep probes in animal brains have shown that the training has produced actual changes in the brain's neurons.[1] Medication can normalize brainwaves only while it is in your system. A ten-year study by Joel Lubar and Associates[2] showed that neurofeedback can effectively change what drugs and therapy often can't.

Brainwaves are reflective of underlying conditions, an expression of neurotransmitter activity. According to Joel Lubar, neurofeedback increases blood flow into the brain. Blood flow, metabolism, and electrical activity all work together to help the brain reset itself in a normal range. When brainwaves are stabilized, symptoms are brought under control. When the problem is slow brainwaves, neurofeedback enables the participant to increase beta frequency and be better able to concentrate. When feedback is used to reduce depression, the person can take more responsibility and function better. When the problem is substance use, the desire for the substance diminishes.

Neurofeedback is actually fun and simple for both children and adults. It is like playing a video game. However, instead of controlling the game with your hands you control the activity with your mind. Each time the brainwaves find their way into the optimal state set by the practitioner, participants are rewarded with positive feedback. This might be in the form of a Pac Man gobbling up his enemy, a car accelerating, or a pleasant tone or image on the computer monitor. The practitioner sets parameters to be challenging but not too difficult, so that participants can move slowly into their optimal brain states. As they learn to control the signals, they are controlling their own brainwave patterns. Just like a video game or physical performance, you start at a level that is fairly easy and gradually increase the challenge as your skills increase.

One of the great advantages of neurofeedback over some other neurological interventions is that it can be tailored to each individual. Brainwaves can be mapped and analyzed for deviations from the norm. For instance, if there is too much theta—which often occurs in brain trauma, depression, and ADHD—and not enough beta, the practitioner will set parameters to increase beta. After approximately twenty sessions, the brain becomes able to find the optimal state on its own without the help of feedback.

One of the pioneers of neurofeedback was Barry Sterman, professor of neurobiology and biobehavioral psychiatry at the UCLA School of Medicine, who in the '70s used a kind of beta wave called sensory motor rhythm (SMR), in the 12 to 15 Hz range to treat epilepsy.[3] His original work was on animals. He found that cats and monkeys could be trained to control their brainwaves.

After Sterman achieved a 60 percent success rate with humans with even the most severe form of epilepsy, experiments were done at other institutions with even higher success rates.

Beta Training[4]

One of Sterman's researchers, Joel Lubar, of the University of Tennessee at Knoxville, noticed that hyperactivity decreased in patients treated for epilepsy; based on this, he created the protocol now used for treatment of ADHD. The protocol is called beta training because ADHD sufferers often show a brainwave pattern with an excess of theta waves (associated with a daydreaming state) and a deficit of betawaves (associated with focus and attention). It makes sense, then, that individuals with ADHD are more detached and less focused. With neurofeedback, those with ADHD learn to inhibit their theta waves and enhance their beta waves. It has been regularly demonstrated that with twenty to thirty sessions, people with ADHD can learn to experience greater clarity of thought and higher energy levels. Over time these changes have been shown to continue even without further treatments. Joel Lubar claims that more than 90 percent of his patients have benefited.

"It Was As If Someone Had Flipped a Switch"

Beta training was where I started my journey with neurofeedback. I was curious about the technology. . . . For a half hour or so, I watched a game: white lines formed in the middle of the highway, and a beep sounded when I produced the right brainwaves. About an hour after that, it was as if someone had flipped a switch. The world looked sharp and crystalline, its colors richer. My thinking was sharper and I had a quiet kind of energy. It lasted a couple of hours.

After five or six sessions, the God-just-painted-the-world effect dissipated, but I noticed other changes. I felt calmer and more centered. I felt more secure in social situations. Particularly important to me was that my mornings were much more productive. I always drink coffee and drag my tail until late morning. Lately I've been getting up, ready to go. By the fifteenth session, the change was unmistakable. As of this writing, it has lasted about a month.

Jim Robbins[5]

Alpha-Theta Protocol[6]

The alpha-theta protocol is very different from beta training. It takes place in the lower registers of the brain's frequencies. The first study of the effectiveness of the alpha-theta protocol on substance abusers was begun in 1982 by Eugene Peniston, a researcher at the Sam Rayburn Memorial Veterans' Center in Bonham, Texas. Peniston hypothesized that alcoholics drink because they cannot get into alpha states naturally, and therefore cannot produce soothing neurotransmitters on their own. He compared ten alcoholics treated with traditional counseling with ten others who had the same counseling plus the alpha-theta training. Peniston claims an 80 percent success rate with those who used the neurofeedback—compared to 20 percent for those receiving traditional treatment.

Memory Training

Scientists from Imperial College, London, and Charing Cross Hospital have announced[7] that they have been able to improve working memory by 10 percent with neurofeedback training. Working memory is a type of memory used to hold and then apply information to perform a task, such as holding a phone number in your mind to recall and use it later. The ability to improve working memory is good news for recovering addicts with memory problems.

We should note here that neurofeedback is not a method for detoxification. You should be through withdrawal before using it. We would also caution you to work with a practitioner who identifies your specific brainwave patterns to determine the type of protocol most appropriate for you.

There are critics of neurofeedback who say that any benefits are due to a placebo effect, but animal studies show that placebo cannot be the primary reason that brainwave biofeedback is effective. Why not? Because placebos do not work on animals. Of course, there is always the possibility of placebo effects in human studies. Expectancy does produce a reaction. But the practitioner can switch around protocols and get different result. (False feedback does not produce the same effect as accurate feedback.) This would not be the case with a placebo effect, because the participant is not able to tell when the practitioner switches protocols and would not respond because of expectation.

Whether you have a specific disorder such as ADHD or just want to improve the functioning of your brain, neurofeedback can be beneficial. When your brain functions better, you will sleep better, you will feel more serene, you will be able to manage your focus and attention, and you will feel more emotionally stable.

Thanks to Dr. Joel Lubar for his contributions to this chapter. For more information on Dr. Lubar and his research refer to his Web site: www.eegfeedback.org.

CHAPTER 9

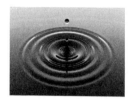

Body Work

THERE ARE A VARIETY OF BODY THERAPIES that you might find beneficial in recovery for natural pain relief, relieving stress, increasing energy, and lifting your mood. Many touch therapies are becoming more and more popular as the benefits become better known. Any of the following methods of balancing or relaxing body tissue can enhance comfort in sobriety.

Therapeutic Massage

Therapeutic massage is used for both relieving pain and reducing stress. In fact, it is based on the idea that there is a relationship between muscle pain and stress; that is, relaxing muscles reduces stress, and reducing stress relaxes muscles. The added benefit is that, when stress responses are lowered, physical disorders, such as high blood pressure and diabetes, improve.

Therapeutic massage—sometimes referred to as Swedish massage—originated about 5,000 years ago in Sweden, thus it's passed the test of time as a way to improve health and well-being.

Reiki and Therapeutic Touch

Reiki and Therapeutic Touch are techniques concerned with moving energy through the body to restore balance. They are based on the idea that there are energy fields within and around the body. These techniques are intended to balance and restore harmony throughout the energy system of the body.

Reiki originated in Japan as a way to bring the mind, body, and spirit into balance. It came from a technique described in Tibetan scriptures almost 3,000 years ago. Therapeutic Touch is the work of Dora Kuntz and Delores Krieger and is influenced by yoga and the Ayurvedic, Tibetan, and Chinese health systems.

With both techniques, there may or may not be physical contact between the therapist and the client, however Reiki is usually a hands-on procedure and therapeutic touch is usually hands off. Therapeutic Touch is usually done with the hand about four inches above the body. It is sometimes said that Reiki allows the energy flow and Therapeutic Touch directs the energy flow.

Therapeutic Touch includes an assessment during which the therapist identifies blockages in energy flow by a feeling of coldness; infection or excess energy by a feeling of warmth; and congestion by variations in sensations experienced. The practitioner works with the client until these areas all feel similar—no area is hotter, colder, or more congested than another. The average treatment lasts about twenty minutes.

Research has discovered that Reiki and therapeutic touch offer similar benefits: relaxation, decreased anxiety, increased sense of well-being, and healing. Both have been found to have a calming effect and to decrease anxiety. When nurses use Therapeutic Touch, patients have been found to need less pain medication.

For more information about Therapeutic Touch call 703-437-4377. For more information about Reiki call the International Center for Reiki Training at 800-332-8112.

Reflexology

Reflexology is a micro-system therapy; that is, various points on the feet are thought to represent various organs and parts of the body. Reflexologists claim that work on these points improves blood flow and energy, thus improving functioning in the corresponding part of the body. Tenderness at a specific site on the foot indicates a potential problem in the associated part of the body. Pressure on that spot leads to unblocked energy.

During a reflexology session, the therapist applies gentle but firm pressure or massage to your feet. Like a good massage, reflexology is very relaxing and is said to lessen anxiety. It is generally safe, but you should still take some precautions. For example, if your feet have been injured in any way, postpone treatment until they've healed. Most reflexologists will not treat you if you have a fever; if you've recently had surgery; if you have blood clots, varicose veins, ulcers, or any other vascular problem in your lower legs; or if you have a pacemaker. So long as you follow these precautions and do not rely on reflexology for any diagnostic purposes, it appears to be a safe way to decrease tension and relieve pain. For more information, call the International Institute of Reflexology at 813-343-4811.

Rolfing

Rolfing, developed by biophysicist Ida Rolf, focuses on the fascia, or connective tissue that binds and connects the body's bones and muscles. Normal fascia is loose, moist, and mobile, allowing muscles and joints to move easily and remain flexible. Chronic stress, injury, and inactivity cause the fascia to thicken and its layers to fuse together.

The purpose of Rolfing is to stretch and unwind the thickened fascia, reestablish proper alignment, restore the normal relationship between bones and muscles, and improve their function. Rolfers claim to be able to reduce pain and spasms, raise your energy levels, improve mood, and make the body more limber, and increase range of motion in the joints. For more information on Rolfing, contact The Rolf Institute of Structural Integration at 800-530-8875.

Myofascial Release

As the name implies, myofascial release also focuses on connective tissue. It is based on the idea that when the myofascia is damaged the constrictions and restrictions interfere with proper functioning throughout the body. When these constrictions are released, there is not only physical relief but also emotional and mental release. Although there are few studies to support myofascial release, it is rapidly becoming more popular, and many who experience it report dramatic outcomes. For more information about this therapy, contact Myofascial Release Treatment Centers at 1-800-FASCIAL.

Merlene: Because I had a daughter-in-law who was a massage therapist that practiced myofascial release, I had heard quite a bit about the therapy's benefits and many stories of astounding outcomes. I had her give me a couple of treatments and then decided to get what is called an intensive—about 100 hours in three weeks—from a therapist in my area. It was an amazing experience. Something happens with myofascial release that I have not heard about with other forms of massage—involuntary movement. The therapist massages one part of the body, and another part moves. I don't mean this is involuntary movement in the sense that I couldn't stop it but in the sense that I didn't consciously initiate it. And I usually did not attempt to stop it because I did not feel at risk in any way. If I did, I could have stopped it. Sometimes it felt as if I had large strands of taffy inside and someone was pulling the taffy on one end causing a response at the point where it was connected at the other end. After I was comfortable with what was happening to me I was able to relax and just let it happen, often entering a very relaxed state in which I had a sense of enlightenment and awareness. At the end of my intensive, I felt better physically, mentally, and spiritually than I can remember feeling since I was a child. I had much more freedom of movement; I felt clean mentally and emotionally; and my energy level was increased.

The Rosen Method

The Rosen Method is a therapy developed by Martha Rosen that combines massage with a form of nondirective counseling. It is based on the idea that traumas and memories are stored in the body as muscular tension. Agitated emotions often result in tense muscles and those emotions can be released through massage. As the massage moves to various areas of the body, the therapist—while monitoring breathing and asking questions—gets the client to talk about potential emotional blocks. The combination of massage and discussion can bring memories and emotions to the surface. Often awareness of the emotion is therapeutic; in other instances, talking about the emotions is helpful. For more information contact The Rosen Institute: 510-845-6606.

Shiatsu

Shiatsu originated in Japan about seventy years ago and is based on Chinese medicine practice. It is considered massage but it is really more a form of acupressure. Like acupuncture, it targets the points where energy flows along meridians throughout the body. It is credited with bringing about the same types of results as acupuncture: primarily pain relief and relaxation.

Craniosacral Therapy

Cerebrospinal fluid bathes the brain and the tissues of the spinal cord. It is prevented from leaking out into the rest of the body by a membrane that encloses the entire nervous system. Cerebrospinal fluid normally flows freely from the head (cranium) to the base of the spine (sacrum). According to craniosacral therapists, this nervous system circulation has a rhythm of its own. They theorize that anything that interrupts the normal flow of cerebrospinal fluid or alters its rhythm and pressure can cause physical and mental problems.

William Sutherland, an osteopath, formulated the theory of craniosacral therapy in the early 1900s. During the last twenty years, his work has been continued and popularized by another osteopathic physician, John Upledger. In the late

1970s, Upledger headed a team of scientists at Michigan State University that produced a model demonstrating the movement of fluid in the nervous system from the head to the tailbone. The researchers concluded that the craniosacral system acts like a semi-closed hydraulic system. Anything that interferes with the flow of spinal fluid flow prevents this movement and raises the pressure on the membranes as well as the tissues of the brain or the spinal cord. This can result in pain from your head to your tail, as well as emotional and behavioral problems.

Craniosacral therapy is intended to relieve the pressure that interferes with the flow of spinal fluid with gentle pressure to the bones of the skull. For more information, contact The Upledger Institute at 800-233-5880.

CHAPTER 10

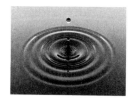

Essential Oil Therapy

FOR THOUSANDS OF YEARS, humankind has benefited from the healing properties of plant oils. Incense and aromatic oils have been used for millennia to enhance religious rituals, to embalm bodies, and to mask unpleasant odors. It wasn't until the 1920s, though, that essential oil therapy became a formal discipline within health care.

Essential oils are aromatic substances extracted from various plant parts, including flowers, roots, bark, leaves, wood resins, and citrus rinds. Essential oils can be sprayed into the air and inhaled, or absorbed through the skin via massage, hot baths, or hot or cold compresses. Some essential oils can be taken internally, but we do not recommend this because a few are toxic when ingested. Essential oils are extracted in concentrated form, but by the time you buy them they have been combined with other carrier oils in order to be used safely.

Essential oils improve your mood and promote good health. Some soothe, some relax, some stimulate and invigorate. They work by reacting with hormones and enzymes after they enter the bloodstream. Essential oils may affect your pulse, blood pressure, or evoke specific memories. For example, clove, rosemary, lavender, and mint stimulate the salivary glands; camphor, calamus, and hyssop are good for the heart and circulation; other aromatics act on the lymphatic, endocrine, nervous, and urinary systems; and bergamot, lavender, and juniper have antiseptic properties, and are said to help a variety of dermatologic disorders when applied to the skin.

"To His Surprise, the Pain and Redness Subsided Very Quickly"

It happened serendipitously when René-Maurice Gattefossé, a French chemist working in the perfume industry, burned his hand very badly. The only "therapy" immediately available to him was a container of pure lavender oil into which he plunged his scorched hand. To his surprise, the pain and redness subsided very quickly, and Gattefossé claimed that the burn healed within hours without leaving a scar. The chemist attributed this salutary effect to the healing and antiseptic properties of the lavender oil. He experimented with several other oils and decided that they, too, had potential for healing a variety of skin disorders. Other French physicians, notably Dr. Jean Valnet, began to use aromatic oils not only for skin problems but for other medical disorders as well, such as anxiety and insomnia. Valnet, who served as an army surgeon during World War II, treated burns and other wounds with essential oils such as clove, thyme, and chamomile. He also found that certain fragrances alleviated some psychiatric problems.

From *Dr. Rosenfeld's Guide to Alternative Medicine*[1]

Calming and comforting oils include sage, sandalwood, patchouli, thyme, jasmine, chamomile, oregano, marjoram, and lavender. Sesquiterpenes, found in the oils of frankincense and sandalwood, help increase the amount of oxygen in the limbic system of the brain, leading to an increase in opioids. Lavender is one of the most popular plants in essential oil therapy. It is known for its relaxing and calming effects, and it is also an excellent remedy for headaches and insomnia. For gentle relaxation, try soaking a towel in warm water infused with lavender. You can re-warm the towel in a microwave and bring the lavender scent to your face and hands to experience this aromatic relaxation.

Invigorating herbal oils include mountain savory, peppermint, spearmint, ginger, citrus, mint, and cardamom. Oils that promote clarity of thought are petitgrain, rosemary, cedarwood, basil, spruce, ginger, fir, bergamot, and clove. Oils that are emotionally healing include cypress, eucalyptus, and wild tansy. Oils that increase spiritual awareness and promote emotional harmony and balance are frankincense, galbanum, grapefruit, melissa, myrrh, yarrow, and juniper. To improve sleep, try chamomile, lavender, or marjoram.

Inhalation

Pleasant aromas can lift your mood, help you sleep, and aid in relaxation. When we inhale a particular scent, it is picked up by two small patches of tissue in the nasal cavity that contain more than 20 million nerve endings that are stimulated by aromas. The scent is converted into a nerve message that is immediately transmitted to the limbic system of the brain, which then relays the aroma to the hypothalamus, triggering both emotional and physiological responses.

A good way to get the most benefit from herbs and flowers is by extracting the essence of the plant by steeping it in water or oil. You can do this yourself using small jars with tight-fitting lids (do not use plastic containers). Place two large handfuls of herbs or flowers in a saucepan. Use a neutrally flavored vegetable oil to cover the herbs or flowers. Heat at a low temperature for twenty to thirty minutes, let the oil cool, strain it into a jar, close tightly, and store in a cool, dark place for up to three weeks. To fill a room with the aroma, place the opened jar on a table. (You can also pour some oil in your bath water or rub it on your body after a bath or shower.)[2]

To prevent inhaling the oil, take care when using a diffuser with essential oil. Certain oils must be used with caution as they are known allergens. Too much of any type of oil might result in an abnormal response. Rosemary appears to have a blood sugar–raising effect. *Eucalyptus citriodora* has been found to have a blood sugar–lowering effect.

Topical Application

Oils can be applied directly to the skin, typically using one to six drops of oil. One to three drops are usually adequate. Oil placed on the feet is rapidly absorbed because of large pores. The ears and the wrists will also rapidly absorb oils. If you are massaging oil onto a large area of the body, dilute the oil by about 30 percent with a neutral-smelling vegetable oil. Don't try to create your own blends of essential oils. Commercial blends are available that have been formulated by people who understand the chemical nature of each oil and how they blend. If mixed improperly, their chemical properties can be altered and you can get an undesirable reaction. It is better to layer individual oils: apply one oil at a time, rub it in, and then apply another oil.

Oils and Water

Essential oils mixed with water can be very pleasing and relaxing. You can fill a water basin with hot water, stir in these essential oils, and lay a towel on top of the water to make a compress. The oils will float to the top, so the towel will absorb the oils in the water. After the towel is completely saturated, wring it out and place it over the area of your body needing the compress. Or you can add three to six drops of oil to your bath water while the tub is filling. Your skin will quickly draw the oil from the top of the water as you soak for about fifteen minutes. Or you can add three to six drops of oil to a half-ounce of bath or shower gel base and add it to your bath water. When showering, you can add three to six drops of oil to a bath or shower gel and apply it to a washcloth.

Raindrop Therapy

Gary Young, of Young Essential Oils, an aromatologist and expert on the art and science of aromatherapy, has developed an application technique called raindrop therapy. This involves dropping oils directly onto the spine from about six inches above the body. The oils are worked into the spine with light strokes that stimulate energy impulses and disperse the oil along the nervous system. This is believed to bring the body into balance. A raindrop massage lasts about forty-five minutes, but the oils continue to work in the body for a week or more following the therapy. Oils used in raindrop therapy are Valor (a blend of rosewood, blue tansy, frankincense, and spruce), thyme, oregano, cypress, birch, basil, peppermint, marjoram, and Aroma Siez (a blend of basil, lavender, cypress, and marjoram).

What Science Says About Essential Oils

Here is what some scientifically valid studies report on the benefits of aromas:

Sleep: In a 1995 report in *The Lancet,* elderly patients who required substantial doses of sleeping pills slept like babies when a lavender aroma was wafted into their bedrooms at night.

Behavior: Mice made hyper-excitable by large amounts of caffeine were calmed by fragrances of lavender, sandalwood, and other oils sprayed into their cages. On the other hand, they became more irritable when exposed to the aroma of orange terpenes, thymol, and certain other substances.

Stress: At Memorial Sloan-Kettering Hospital in New York, after exposure to the aroma of vanilla, patients reported that they were 63 percent less claustrophobic. The patients' anxiety may have been lessened by the intensity of the pleasant memories evoked by the vanilla aroma. In another study of 122 patients under obvious stress in an intensive care unit, patients felt much better when they were given aromatherapy with oil of lavender than when they simply rested or had a massage.

Isadore Rosenfeld, MD[3]

Vita Flex Therapy

Vita Flex Therapy, part of a system developed by Stanley Burroughs, uses the reflex system of the body to release tension. It combines using essential oils with a form of massage similar to reflexology for the whole body. Applied with rotation hand movements, the massage releases healing energy along the neuro-electrical pathways. Healing energy is created by the contact between the fingertips and contact points. The resulting energy follows the neuro-pathways of the nervous system to points where there is a break in the electrical circuit. This technique is believed to have originated in Tibet, many thousands of years ago, before acupuncture was discovered. Vita Flex therapists say this is a superior form of reflexology. Although it utilizes the same principles, Vita Flex produces less discomfort than traditional reflexology. In addition, there are 5,000 identified Vita Flex points in the body, compared to 365 acupuncture points used in reflexology. Combining the electrical energy with the healing properties of essential oils releases healing power, relieving tension, drowsiness, weariness, and discomfort. Oils used in Vita Flex Therapy are Valor and White Angelica (a blend of ylang ylang, rose, angelica, melissa, sandalwood, geranium, spruce, myrrh, hyssop, bergamot, and rosewood).

If you're considering essential oil therapy, or are already using it, there are certain cautions you should take. According to Isadore Rosenfeld, MD:

- Aromatic oils vary in quality, and their production is not regulated, so make sure your source is reliable. Always ask for the purest available brand.
- Do not consume aromatic oils. Some can be toxic.
- Store aromatic oils in a cool place. Some, such as jasmine and neroli, should be refrigerated. Most oils retain their potency for two to three years, but citrus oils lose their potency within a year.
- With the exception of topical lavender oil for burns or insect bites, never use concentrated, undiluted oil. Refer to a good book on aromatherapy for instructions on diluting oil.
- If your skin is sensitive, always apply a very small amount of the diluted oil before you try the whole treatment, to make sure you're not allergic to it. Five percent of the population

reacts adversely to aromatic oils.

- Keep all aromatic oils away from children.
- Always close your eyes when inhaling aromatic oil. The vapors can be irritating at close range. Don't apply any oils close to your eyes.
- Do not use mint oils at night—they can cause insomnia.
- Avoid oils of sweet fennel and rosemary if you have epilepsy. These substances may increase the excitability of the brain and induce seizures.
- If you're pregnant, avoid oils of arnica, basil, clary sage, cypress, juniper, myrrh, sage, and thyme. Some obstetricians believe that these oils can cause the uterus to contract. A woman who is at risk of a miscarriage, or who has abnormal bleeding, should keep away from chamomile and lavender. If the doctor approves, a pregnant woman may use diluted oils of peppermint, rose, and rosemary after the fourth month.
- People with high blood pressure should avoid oils of rosemary, sage, and thyme.

For more information or to order essential oils, call Young Living at 800-371-3515.

CHAPTER 11

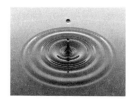

Support People

A SUCCESSFUL RECOVERY INVOLVES developing new and more meaningful social networks. That means finding resources and making contacts that will enable you to meet new people who can offer more than just drinking company. As you replace drug use with meaningful, enduring values and activities, you will want to associate with people who share those values.

They say in AA that to find sobriety you must change playgrounds and playmates. The people you associated with while using are tied to your addiction-based lifestyle. It is not that they are bad; you just have one central thing in common with them—your use of mood-altering substances. If you choose to spend most of your time around old using buddies, ignoring their expectations for you to use chemicals can become stressful or even impossible.

As for the playgrounds, it has been said that no one frequents a house of ill repute to listen to the piano player. By the same token, you do not go to a bar to have orange juice. It is not just a question of not associating with your old friends or not frequenting your old hangouts. It is more a question of what new places you are going to and what new friends you are meeting. Your playgrounds will change automatically as you meet new sober people.

Being a social animal is different from being a party animal. Becoming social is an art; being a party animal is nothing more than getting high or drunk, laughing a lot, acting crazy, and not remembering what you did or said. Reorienting your lifestyle around new values is an essential part of recovery. The values that allowed you to keep using will not allow you to stay sober. A lifestyle conducive to using is not conducive to sobriety. Friends who encourage drinking or using do not usually encourage abstinence. Places where it was easy to drink or use are not usually places where it is easy not to. New friends, new activities, and new social contacts are part of recovery.

Mutual-Help Groups

A mutual-help group is a valuable source for establishing or reestablishing a meaningful social network. You will find people that understand not only your struggles but your need for deeper and more meaningful relationships. They will offer you friendship, support, acceptance, and encouragement. They provide fun activities without alcohol or other drugs. Don't forget how important it is to learn to have fun—with people who do not center their good times around mood-altering chemicals.

In recovery, you need the support of others, especially the support of people with the same condition. For those who have problems relating to the principles or practices of twelve-step groups there are other support groups available. Most groups—whether twelve step or another group—encourage a new way of life based on honesty and reaching out to others. They offer a means for making the right changes at the right time. They are based on members sharing their experiences and what has worked for them. These groups are places where you can meet people with whom you can feel safe and comfortable in new and healthy ways as you attempt to understand the disorder you have and share with those in the same boat.

Alcoholics Anonymous

The most well-known support group is Alcoholics Anonymous (AA), founded in the 1930s by people who had tried many other methods of abstaining from alcohol and had failed. They found that mutual support enabled them to do what had previously been unattainable. AA has endured over the years, and its principles apply to other twelve-step programs such as Narcotics Anonymous, Overeaters Anonymous, Cocaine Anonymous, and Gamblers Anonymous.

AA is especially helpful for individuals who prefer a spiritually-based group. The steps of AA are spiritual principles. AA encourages you to accept the help of a higher power, though that power can be defined as you choose. It can even be the power of the group itself.

AA offers the recovering person much that professional treatment cannot offer. It offers a readily available environment that is conducive to ongoing recovery and sobriety. AA is available twenty-four hours a day in every major city around the world. You are never farther away from a meeting than the telephone. In large metropolitan areas, meetings are held at all times of the day and night. You can always have the phone number of someone who will help you avoid that one drinking or drug episode.

AA doesn't cost anything except time, energy, and a motivation to stop drinking or using. You need a place to go to meet other people who want to have fun and socialize without drugs or alcohol. Many recovering people begin rebuilding their social life with friends and acquaintances they find at meetings.

Rational Recovery

Rational recovery (RR) is an alternative support program utilized primarily by people who are uncomfortable with the spiritual nature of Alcoholics Anonymous. As the name implies, RR is based on the concepts of rational thinking. It was started by Jack Trimpey using the principles of rational-emotive therapy developed by Albert Ellis. In rational recovery, you learn to be aware of your emotions and where they come from. You learn to recognize that emotions are not forced upon you by others or by outside situations. They are your own response to situations, and you can learn to control your response. Rational recovery suggests the five-point criteria developed by Maxie Maultsby to evaluate a thought to determine whether it is logical.

1. If I believe this thought to be true, will it help me remain sober, safe, and alive?
2. Is this thought objectively true, and upon what evidence am I forming this opinion?
3. Is this thought producing feelings I want to have?
4. Is this thought helping me reach a chosen goal?
5. Is this thought likely to minimize conflict with others?

Rational recovery helps you identify irrational ideas and beliefs that perpetuate addictive behavior and then provides the means to change your emotions and behavior.[1]

An AA Sponsor

The principles of AA are simple, but at first they can be misunderstood. Therefore, a practice has developed whereby experienced members program make themselves available to newer members as a sponsor. A sponsor's responsibility is to provide support during recovery, answer questions, discuss the various aspects of the program, assist the new members in identifying meetings that meet their needs, and direct them to appropriate literature and resources that they may need to fully understand the program.

AA sponsors are not therapists or counselors, nor are they responsible for telling other members how to work their programs. All members are responsible for interpreting the principles for themselves and developing their own programs based on those principles. The sponsor is merely a sounding board, a supportive friend, and a knowledgeable resource.

Counseling

If you started drinking or using drugs early in life, you may have skipped some developmental stages of growth. The teens and early twenties are years when emotional and social maturation take place. If drinking and drug use occur during that time, that developmental process may not occur or it may be retarded.

At whatever point you decide to give up drug or alcohol use as a way of coping with life, counseling can aid you in the process of learning to manage your emotions and developing the insights and self-awareness that you may have missed by addictive living.

A counselor can help you resolve the pervasive shame that may affect your recovery. Addiction is often accompanied by shame for a number of reasons. First you may feel shame because of a condition that existed before your addiction (such as ADHD) and which increased your vulnerability for using mood-altering substances. Second, you may have done things while drinking or using drugs that you would not do sober and which are very shameful to you now. Third, you may have a history of repeated relapse that you and other people interpret as being weak willed or lacking strength of character. (Actually, the fact that you have kept trying despite what has been perceived as failure shows strong will and strength of character.) And fourth, there is the stigma that accompanies addiction. Our society views addiction as a shameful condition. Even though we live in a culture that encourages drinking, overeating, pill popping, and other excesses, when a person becomes addicted to alcohol, pills, food, or gambling, they are looked upon as morally lacking, self-centered, pleasure-obsessed individuals. Learning to accept yourself as a person of worth despite the burden of shame that you or society has placed upon you can be a positive outcome of counseling. A counselor can help you replace misperceptions you may have about yourself, the world, or your addiction with accurate perceptions that facilitate behavior change.

In recovery you may need to learn or relearn certain life skills. If you want to change your behavior, a counselor can help. You have developed many skills that have helped you survive addiction. These same skills can be modified to help you live sober.

David: I am a reality therapist. I like reality therapy (RT) because it is a very simple approach to helping you change your behavior. It asks you some direct questions to help you evaluate what you are doing and help you make plans to change what you are doing if you really want to change. The questions are: What are you doing now? Is that working for you? If not, what are you going to do instead? The idea is to figure out what is not working in your life and not just eliminate it but replace it with a better chosen behavior. With RT you take small, manageable steps that lead you where you want to go.

Coaching

Coaching is not counseling. Coaching is a term taken from sports that refers to an alliance that empowers success. Coaching is now being used to empower professional success, educational success, and personal success. ADHD coaching is being used extensively by people with attention deficit hyperactivity disorder. We recommend ADHD-type coaching for people recovering from addiction. In the first place, many of you who have had problems with addiction also have attention deficit disorder, treated or untreated. Second, people in sobriety experience many of the symptoms of ADHD. Third, and most important, many skills that people with ADHD need to develop are lacking in those with addictions.

The purpose of any coaching is to enhance performance. The purpose of ADHD coaching is to enable you to enhance performance by helping you (1) set goals, (2) devise a plan for reaching your goals, (3) set priorities, (4) make decisions, and (5) keep on track. A coach offers guidance and support while giving responsibility to you. The first phase in the coaching process is setting the agenda—identifying your long-term goals. And remember, this is your agenda, not the coach's agenda. The second phase is making short-term goals that will meet day-to-day needs and help you achieve your long-term goals. During the second phase, it is important to review your progress to determine if the long-term goals are still applicable.

The value of coaching is having someone available to guide you when you find it difficult to sort things out and prioritize tasks. Someone trained to do so can help you keep on track by continually holding up your goals and identifying whether your actions will achieve your goals. The coach can help you keep moving when you feel paralyzed by the obstacles you encounter as you face the problems created by your addiction. The coach can also help you identify what supports need to be put in place to increase your chances for success, determine what you want or need to accomplish between coaching sessions, and decide what tasks will help you accomplish those things. When you and the coach determine what skills are lacking that prevent you from achieving your goals you will make plans for developing those skills or change your goals according to the skills you already have. The greatest value of having a coach is having someone to provide regular reminders of where you want to go and what you need to do to get there.

Coaching differs from counseling in that the power lies not in the coach or the client, but in the coaching alliance. The client is a full partner in the alliance. The coach's goal is always to facilitate the client's agenda. By asking powerful and direct questions, reminding you of your agenda, and keeping you focused, the coach allows you to plan your own course and take the steps to keep you on it. The alliance provides a safe environment for you to practice developing life skills. The phone number for the American Coaching Association is 610-825-8572.

CHAPTER 12

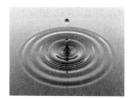

Stress-Reducing Activities

STRESS AFFECTS YOUR BODY AND YOUR MIND. It affects your thinking, feelings, memory, sleep patterns, daily functioning, and physical and mental health. When a sudden alert is sounded in the body, the center part of the brain, or the hypothalamus, sends a message to the adrenal gland to release cortisol. Cortisol increases the heart rate, increases the blood pressure, and releases stored glucose from the liver and muscle cells into the bloodstream for quick energy.

Some stress in life is necessary. It keeps you functioning. Without some stress you would not take care of yourself, go to work, or do anything for your family. But too much stress is harmful. Each of us has a level of stress at which we function most effectively. Your best stress level is high enough to keep you productive, yet low enough not to hurt you or the people around you. Finding the level of stress that is useful without being destructive is important for your recovery from addiction. You can relapse because of too little stress (no constructive concern about your addiction) or because of too much stress (which produces excessive worry and anxiety).

One of the most agonizing chronic abstinence symptoms is stress sensitivity. Most recovering people have a low stress tolerance and overreact to stress. As we have discussed before, this can sabotage even the best efforts at sobriety. We have talked about foods and supplements and environmental changes to reduce stress levels. There are also actions you can take to reduce stress and increase serenity and peace of mind. The relaxation response (the decrease of blood pressure and pulse rate and the improved utilization of oxygen) occurs because of what you do and think. You can learn to relax.

Deep Relaxation

You are probably aware that your muscles cannot relax and tense at the same time. You can learn to relax your muscles when you choose, thereby reducing tension. You can also learn to form pictures in your mind that help you relax. And you can learn to talk to yourself in a way that reduces tension and increases your feelings of comfort and well-being.

Deep relaxation allows the body and mind to reduce stress and produce a sense of wellbeing. What occurs when you relax is the opposite of what is called the fight or flight response. When you relax, your muscles become heavy, your body temperature rises, and your breathing and heart rate slow down.

To experience deep relaxation, create a quiet place for yourself. Separate yourself from the world in your quiet place. Lie on your back or sit in a comfortable chair with your feet on the floor. Close your eyes, release distracting thoughts, try to put background noises and sounds out of your thoughts.

Breathe deeply and relax your body. You do not make your body relax—you allow it to relax. You focus your concentration on one thing and allow distractions to drift from your awareness.

With some relaxation methods, the focus is on the physical states you are trying to change (your muscles, body temperature, breathing, or heartbeat). With other methods, you do not concentrate on your physical state, but on a color, a sound, a word or mantra, or a mental image.

If you choose to focus on physical states, begin with your muscles. Allow them to become heavy. Then concentrate on raising your temperature. You can do this by sensing a spot of heat in your forehead or chest and allowing it to flow throughout your body. Then think about your breathing. Let it become slower and slower. Breathe from your abdomen, rather than your chest. Then feel your heartbeat and concentrate on slowing it down.

If you choose to relax by concentrating on something other than your physical state, you can think of a color. Concentrate on that color, fill your mind with that color, become a part of that color. Or feel yourself in motion, floating, tumbling, and rolling. Or repeat a pleasant word over and over to yourself. Or imagine yourself in a soothing place, such as by a quiet lake, in a green meadow, or in a beautiful garden. These are relaxation exercises you can do by yourself without the aid of a book or a tape.

Numerous books and tapes are available to guide you through the relaxation process. Or you can record a tape yourself and play it when you want to relax. Deep relaxation reduces your stress and helps you feel better. Relaxation exercises can help you manage chronic abstinence symptoms and heal your addicted brain.

Breathing

Deep breathing aids in relaxation. In his newsletter, "Self-Healing," Dr. Andrew Weil has noted that deep breathing has been shown to lower blood pressure, decrease or stop heart arrhythmias, improve digestion, increase blood circulation, decrease anxiety, and improve the quality of sleep. To distinguish deep breathing from shallow breathing, pay attention to your chest and your abdomen. Chest breathing is usually shallow breathing; abdominal breathing is usually deep breathing.

Dr. Weil describes a yoga-style method of breathing like this:

Start by sitting with your back straight or lying in a comfortable position. Place the tip of your tongue to the ridge in back of your upper front teeth and keep it there during the entire exercise. Exhale through the mouth with a whoosh sound. Close your mouth and inhale through your nose to the count of four. Hold your breath for seven counts and then exhale, with the whoosh sound, to the count of eight. Do this for four cycles.

There is a connection between your breathing and your emotional state. Fear, anger, and frustration restrict breathing. Restricted breathing increases negative emotional states. Your sense of well-being can be enhanced by your breathing. When you calm your breath you calm your mind. Calming your breathing throughout the day brings a sense of peacefulness. The constitution of the blood is altered through oxygen exchange which, in turn, leads to more relaxed breathing. Here is another deep breathing exercise you can try:

1. While sitting or lying down, place your hands on your stomach and chest.
2. Sigh (audibly) several times.

3. Slowly and fully inhale through the mouth, filling your lungs comfortably from the bottom to the top. Imagine you are bringing energy into your body.
4. Without hesitation, exhale through your nose, emptying your lungs from the top to the bottom comfortably. Visualize yourself releasing your tensions as you breathe out.
5. Repeat this procedure for ten to fifteen minutes, until you are totally and pleasantly absorbed with the breathing process and alert but not focusing on any other thoughts or activities. There will be a feeling of peace and serenity just in controlling your breathing process.

Yoga

Developed over centuries, yoga is used to reduce stress, improve flexibility, and provide mental clarity. Yoga is a technique with three major components: posture, breathing, and meditation. The first objective of yoga is to maintain one of a variety of yoga poses for a specified period of time. The ultimate goal is to gain the self control needed for proper breathing and for effective meditation. The breathing exercises consist of a routine in which the lungs are filled with air that is held and then released.

The goal of the meditation component is to detach from your environment and to experience peace, enlightenment, and tranquility.

Here is a scaled-down version of yoga that you can follow easily and effectively, as described in the "Lifetime Health Letter"[1] from the University of Texas—Houston.

- *For exercise:* Sit forward in a chair, your feet flat on the floor. Put your right hand on your left knee. With your left hand, hold the back of the chair. Look straight ahead, inhale, and then as you slowly exhale, turn to your left. Pull with both hands to rotate your spine as much as possible without strain. Hold the rotated position for a few seconds, continuing to breathe easily. Return to the forward position. Then, put your left hand on your right knee, and repeat the steps, twisting to the right.

- *For breathing:* Sit straight with both hands flat against your stomach, just below the navel. Relax your stomach and allow it to push out as you inhale. Then, as you exhale, tighten your stomach and flatten your back. Concentrate on the sound your breath makes in the back of your throat. Breathe smoothly and steadily through your nose; don't hold your breath at any time. Repeat this procedure several times.

- *For meditation:* Sit quietly and comfortably in a chair or on the floor. Close your eyes and take a few full, deep breaths. Concentrate on the sound you make when you breathe in and out. Relax your breath and, at the same time, consciously relax your facial muscles. Progressively relax the rest of your body, beginning with the shoulders and arms, working your way down to your feet. Become limp without slouching. Try to be completely silent, inside and out. Imagine a pleasant scene to help yourself achieve total relaxation. After a few minutes, begin to breathe more deeply; then stretch your arms and imagine your energy being totally renewed.

Several scientific reports suggest that yoga can reduce blood pressure and heart rate and improve circulation, as well as help you relax, ease chronic pain, and improve your memory and concentration. Some of these benefits may be due to a release of opioids.

Contact the International Association of Yoga Therapists, 415-383-4587 for the name of a yogi in your area.

Sleep

Sleep is an important ingredient of good health. Because of your addictive lifestyle, you may have developed poor sleep habits. In addition, you may experience abstinence-related sleep problems. This may be especially true if you have used alcohol excessively in the past. Although alcohol is sedating, it disrupts normal sleep patterns and deprives you of REM sleep (dream sleep). When you are no longer drinking, there is a rebound effect in which your body tries to catch up on lost REM sleep and, for a period of time, you may experience an excessive amount of disturbing dreams.

To enhance the quality of recovery, you may need to enhance the quality and quantity of sleep. The following are some general considerations are:

- Be sure the temperature of the room is comfortable for you. Wear socks to bed if you have cold feet.
- Maintain regular sleeping times by going to sleep and awakening at the same time each day.
- Avoid exercising close to bedtime. Exercise is a stimulant and can disturb your sleep.
- Avoid stimulants such as caffeine (or tyrosine) near bedtime.
- Take a warm bath or shower close to bedtime.
- Begin to relax and wind down beginning two hours before bedtime: Listen to music. Do relaxation exercises. Read.
- Eat a high complex carbohydrate dinner with little or no protein.
- Eat a high-tryptophan bedtime snack.
- Choose your mattress and pillows carefully. Make sure your weight is evenly distributed. Make sure your pillow provides enough support for your neck.
- Maintain a quiet bedroom without bright lights.

Physical Exercise

We have a friend who used to say, "I have a theory that exercise causes cancer. The only thing I exercise is caution. I only enjoy long walks when they are taken by people who nag me to exercise." She was kidding, of course, but behind the humor she was saying something many people would like to say, "We would like a good excuse not to exercise and any good theory will do." The interesting thing we want you to know is that our friend has discovered that she is diabetic and, following her doctor's direction, began walking every day. She had to start gradually and work up. She now walks two miles every day and, in addition to helping her control her diabetes, her walk has become a high point of her day. She will readily tell you how beneficial exercise is and how much it has helped her not just physically but mentally.

Our purpose here is not to convince you that you should endure the physical pain of exercise to reap the gain. It is to encourage you to establish an exercise program in order to relieve the pain you may already be experiencing. The whole purpose of this book is to provide options for increasing pleasure, not pain, in sobriety. We are not going to discuss the benefits of exercise on your heart or lungs or for weight loss. You probably already know how important exercise is for your general health. Our purpose is to remind you of the benefits in reducing your stress by changing your brain chemistry. Certainly, exercise is important to your physical health. What we want to offer you is the pleasure reward that you can get from physical movement.

The truth is that physical activity can be fun, stimulating, and relaxing. A good exercise plan can add pleasure instead of pain to your life. The trick is finding a physical activity that is right for you, something you enjoy doing. No one sticks to an exercise program that is not enjoyable.

To Be Alive Is to Be Moving

"The unmoving water becomes the stagnant pool. The moving body freely channels the energy of life. Moving encourages movement. The more you move, the better you move. Energy creates energy—in a continuous, circling process—in a constant dance. Exercise makes us feel good—not just physically, but emotionally and spiritually. As if the physical advantages of exercise were not enough, its connection to the ways we think and feel about ourselves is remarkable. The moving body is the body releasing stress, letting go of pent-up emotions and unblocking channels for energy."

From *The Wellness Workbook*[3]

The more we move, the better we feel, the more motivated we are to move, and the more energy we have. We feel enlivened when we move. Movement allows us to feel our muscles work, our heart beat, and the blood flow through our bodies, creating energy and a feeling of well-being.

Many recovering people have found exercise to be extremely helpful in freeing them from the limitations of chronic abstinence symptoms. We know many recovering addicts who stop in the middle of their day's activities to exercise when they are feeling anxious or having difficulty concentrating or remembering. After exercising they feel much better and are more productive (and easier to get along with). Researchers at the University of North Carolina—Greensboro found that aerobic exercise reduces depression and anxiety levels in alcoholics.

Research indicates that exercise actually neutralizes brain chemicals that otherwise would increase craving for mood-altering substances. According to the National Center for Health

Statistics, frequent exercisers have higher levels of endorphins and demonstrate more positive moods and less anxiety than those who exercise too little or not at all.

David: Different forms of exercise have different payoffs for me. I have chosen these forms of exercise as strengthening contributions to my sobriety. Hiking or taking a long vigorous walk gives me special time to be completely alone with myself and my God, to meditate and to pray.

I find that movement of my body up hills and down inclines in the heart of nature allows me to think more clearly, often resolving issues or making short-range plans. I find that a walk enables me to break out of the dull stupor that daily routine can bring. Because I automatically feel good while walking, my awareness of my surroundings is also sharpened as if a newly discovered sense is emerging. I then begin to think in a more positive way about myself and my life. I feel more in control of my life. By the end of the walk I am ready to meet new challenges with a new sense of inner strength.

Tennis relaxes me in another way. It provides strenuous exercise with almost every muscle being used with complete awareness of my physical self. It feels good to reach out and slam the ball, providing a surge of power and energy and anger release.

Fellowship with my partner is also healthy and relaxing for me. Even though we are competing, it is all in fun. There is laughing, yelling, and just plain letting go.

Swimming is my special activity. I know of no other recreation that allows me more feelings of surrender. When I let go and become part of the water, I seem to flow through it with my worries and tension dissolving. Exercise is a vital part of my sobriety program and improves the quality of my life.

Aerobic Exercise

Regular exercise in which we use the whole body and keep moving at a steady pace—dancing, jogging, walking, swimming, bicycling—is aerobic and not only relieves stress and gives us a lift, but burns fat. Aerobic exercise increases oxygen intake. Increasing oxygen increases endorphins. While we do not recommend that you limit yourself to aerobic exercise, we strongly recommend that you participate in some aerobic activity every day. It is a good idea to have a variety of activities from which to choose so that an exercise plan is not dependent on partners or on the weather.

Walking is an excellent form of aerobic exercise that is available to anybody. Walking can reduce tension and anxiety immediately. It is one of the most efficient forms of exercise and can be done safely throughout your life. It is also inexpensive and does not require special equipment other than good shoes. It offers the extra benefit of giving you time to reflect and organize your thoughts.

Walking can easily be incorporated into your daily activity. Maybe you can walk to work or to the bank, post office, or to visit a friend. Try taking the stairs instead of an elevator. Walk around the airport while waiting for your plane.

Stretching

Stretching exercises for warming up and cooling down will make your body more flexible. We recommend that you use stretching exercises throughout your day to relax muscles, reduce stiffness, and ease tension.

It is especially helpful to relax the muscles of your neck and shoulders throughout the day. Many people store a lot of tension in this area. Raise both of your shoulders at the same time and slowly rotate them in a circle, backward and then forward. Then roll your head around several times in a full circle as you keep your back straight.

Another place that many people store tension is in the lower back. To strengthen and relax those muscles, lie on your back with knees bent and feet flat on the floor. Tighten your abdominal muscles, grip your buttocks together, and flatten your lower back against the floor. Repeat this several times. Then bring one leg toward your chest. Pull the leg to your chest with your hands. Slowly curl your head toward your bent knee and hold for a count of five. Repeat the exercise with the other leg. Then do the exercise with both legs simultaneously. If you do these exercises for a few minutes every day, you will prevent or reduce much strain in your lower back.

Stress-Relief Tip

For a short tension reliever and also to improve circulation to the extremities, including the head, try placing the palms of your hands on your eyes for a few minutes. Follow this by placing your hands on the back of your head and twisting your body right and left while still seated. While your hands are still placed on the back of your head, touch each elbow to the knee on the same side and then back into the resting position.

Now, place one hand up and over behind your head, touching your back, and place the other hand on the opposite elbow and stretch. Alternately, bend the knees to the chest, one at a time, while sitting on a chair. Next, stretch by placing your feet and hands as far back on each side of the chair as you are able. Complete this exercise with a moment of relaxation by again placing your palms on your eyes and breathing deeply.

Diana W. Guthrie[3]

Fun, Laughter, and Play

Fun is a necessary part of life and of recovery, and it is often neglected. It is not only a part of recovery; it is an essential ingredient of life. Learning to enjoy life naturally will take time and practice because in the past fun has occurred unnaturally through mind-altering chemicals. So it will take some time to convince yourself that you do have the ability to have fun, to enjoy and celebrate without altering your mood artificially. You have the ability to create pleasure in natural ways. Fun and laughter relate directly to the production of opioids. Fun is first and foremost a change of attitude, reaction, and perception about yourself as you slow down and experience life in the present.

Play is usually perceived as something separate and apart from life. Fun is seen as the icing of life; as long as you get your work done you can then, and only then, have fun. Life should be fun and fun a priority, not something we do when and if we have time. We can become so serious about eating right and getting regular exercise that we never allow ourselves to have fun. Life without fun is like a long dental appointment.

From time to time take breaks in your schedule that add color, spontaneity, and some zaniness to life. Put on your favorite music, sing, dance around the room, and let the child in you out. Have a water fight. Make yourself up like a clown. Get silly with the one you love. See what you can think of that is a little crazy and a lot of fun. Find people that you can have fun with; people that can let go and try new things.

Do you ever watch children having fun? They do not make a distinction between work and play. Play is their work. They play when they walk, talk, or when they are putting together puzzles. They are constantly using their developing senses to explore this new world and, for the most part, are happy with their exploration. Don't let society's messages to act your age or grow up or stop being foolish deprive you of the richness of life that play offers.

You may be so programmed to believe that playing is wasting time that you need permission to play. Well, we give you permission. You must play for your health, your well-being, and your recovery. You will find that you are able to accomplish more if you take time for play than if you neglect it. We can learn about play from children. Observe how they give themselves to each moment, allowing them to enjoy and experience whatever they are doing.

Fun is its own reward. Fun feels good, and it enables us to feel good about ourselves.

True enjoyment is characterized by laughter. Laughter releases feel-good brain chemicals and lightens our hearts. After we laugh we feel better, we think better, and we function better. Humor helps us adapt to change. Recovery requires a lot of change. Why not make it easier on yourself by seeing the humor and learning to laugh at yourself? Laughing at yourself allows you to give yourself permission to be imperfect. And when you can find humor in your own imperfections, it is easier to accept imperfections in others.

Research shows that laughter increases creativity and the ability to mentally organize information. Studies also show that humor, laughter, or mild elation enables people to remember, make decisions, and figure things out better. It seems this feel-good stuff is just what a person with chronic abstinence symptoms needs. Lighten up. Laugh a lot. It can only do you good.

Laughter is life's shock absorber. It allows you to take yourself lightly while taking other things seriously. Laughter is internal jogging, and you don't have to get dressed to do it.

At Play
by David

Come, child, blend with me.
The time is now, as only time can be.
Come, child, let me share your world where pain is a stranger,
and glances laced with sweet innocence,
dance on a world made just for you.

Come, child, let me into your eyes.
Share your world where time has no back or front,
just a middle where all is now
as you contemplate some beauty of nature
cast in this plant or that bug.
Come, child, I will honor this time
where we may touch this now together,
as I learn of your wisdom
that I passed so blindly by on the path to "adult."

Come, child, allow me into your joyful laughter—
that clean innocent music where love and joy were born.
Come, child, remind me through your dancing eyes
of when I, too, was eternal and praised the world
through uncluttered observations, never mindful or
caring of expectations the world was casting my way,
dulling my senses through its call to sameness,
where wrong is to be different, where it's wrong to be me.

Come, child, teach me your ways once again
and allow me into your space to rest,
to find forgotten fragments of my self,
to reacquaint myself with the magic moment,
to be all that I can be—here and now.

Children and Laughter: The Best Medicine

Look for things all around you to laugh about. We keep a notebook of funny things children in our family have said. Here are some favorites:

- My teeth are shivering.
- God made me an eating person.
- You plug it in, and I'll plug it out.
- Why are you sleeping with your breakfast? (To someone eating in bed)
- I need a couple of water.
- A ghost is hollow on the inside and doesn't have any shell on the outside.
- Don't call Mom the old lady. She's no lady.
- Sometimes I snore when I laugh.
- Trix are for folks, too. You can have some; you're a folk.

Consider this old Japanese proverb, "Time spent laughing is time spent with the gods." Garrison Keillor says it this way. "Humor is not a trick. Humor is a presence in the world . . . like grace . . . and shines on everybody."

The Clown Chakra

The Clown Scientists have found that all our problems can be placed under one heading: "Seriousness." Seriousness is the leading cause of everything from cancer to reincarnation.

Scientists from the Clown Academy have already discovered a new source of healing. It is a psychic energy point located between the heart chakra and the throat chakra. It is called the Clown Chakra.

If people are feeling miserable, if they have financial problems, if their relationship situation is the pits, if they are in ill health, if they have a need to sue people, if they find fault with their brother, then obviously, their Clown Chakra is closed.

When this happens, the scientists have observed under a high-powered microscope that the cells of every organ display a sad face, and, when the Clown Chakra is open and functioning normally, the cells display a happy face.

The scientists realized that, if a person is ill, it is because his mind has projected guilt onto the cells of his body and has forced out the love that is normally found within each cell of the body. The cells are therefore saying, "I Lack Love," or "ILL" for short.

The scientists also discovered that all disease is due to the fact that the cells are out of ease, or dis-eased.

When the Clown Chakra is opened and working (or rather, playing) properly, the psychic mechanism sucks up misery, pain, anger, resentment, grievances, unhappiness, etc., and converts the energy into tiny red heart-shaped balloons. The red heart-shaped balloons contain Love and Joy.

These balloons are directed to the dis-eased cell or situation, and a happy face appears instantly. When the light enters the darkness, the darkness is gone. Sometimes these red heart-shaped balloons are called endorphins, due to the fact that, when anyone experiences them, the feeling of separation ends. They experience being back home with All That Is and hence are no longer an orphan. This is the well-known end-orphan (endorphin) effect.

So, if you think someone is attacking you, Clown Scientists recommend that you visualize sending that person red heart-shaped balloons filled with love and joy. Remember to keep your Clown Chakra open and remember to laugh.

Pets

It is well-documented that pets can improve our health. Studies have shown that our enjoyment of our pets raises our spirits, lowers our blood pressure and cholesterol, and overall just makes life more enjoyable. Their unique, unconditional relationship with us helps us feel appreciated and important.

Did Someone Mention Pets?

Did you ask about Sammy? Well, since you ask, we just happen to have pictures. He is our seven-pound Papillion who we named Samson because he hasn't the faintest idea he isn't a Great Dane. He keeps us laughing with his antics: trying to cram a ball and a bone in his mouth at the same time, trying to jump up on a bed with a toy bigger than he is, or carrying around an empty plastic bottle big enough for him to climb into. He just doesn't know limits. What Sam lacks in weight he makes up for in determination and speed. Just when you think he's in another room, there he is, right on your heels. Like the speed of light. What Sammy is really big on, though, is heart. It's hard to believe so much love and affection can reside in so small a creature. He always wants to be where we are. They say if you like to go to the bathroom alone, don't get a Papillion. Sammy will sit at the door and wait for you to come out. When anyone comes to the house, he gets extremely excited. We haven't told him that not everyone who comes to the door comes to see him. He gets so excited he gets the zoomies, zipping around and around the house like he is propelled by a motor. Sammy's special gift is touching. He not only wants to be in the same room with us at all times, he wants to be as close as he can get. He must sleep with us, usually snuggled up against a leg or a butt, kind of like a furry Fixodent. As soon as we stir in the morning, he smothers us with hugs and kisses. He hugs by putting his front paws on our chests and snuggling his face into our necks. Of course, you know what his kisses are, and he always overdoes it, not just with us, but with anyone who can't escape. He just can't hold his licker. Since he has come into our lives, sleep has been more restful, laughter more frequent, and every day brighter. Some people say we are a little overzealous and spoil him a bit. One friend says in his next life he wants to come back as Sammy. But most people who meet him admit that Sammy lights up the place.

Softening the Environment

Overload, high distractibility, hyper-vigilance, and stimulus augmentation all mean principally the same thing. When a person's filtering system does not work well, perception is altered. But you can learn to soften your environment and separate yourself periodically from unpleasant noises and sensations.

David: I may leave home without my American Express card. But I will never leave home without my earplugs! One of the best gifts of my life was a pair of earplugs given to me by a friend that works for General Motors. They have ridges on them that fit comfortably and snugly into the ear and, best of all, they work great. I can still hear with them in, but they soften the noise quite a bit so at least my nervous system doesn't spasm when that no-muffler car roars by.

In addition to earplugs, a white-noise machine might be helpful. These wonderful little gadgets emit a soft, masking sound like a waterfall, an ocean, or similar sound that covers up those clanging, banging noises. A fan or a computer may work because they both emit white noise of their own. Some people leave on the fan to their central air or heat to give them constant white noise. Many of us are truly fans of fans.

You can also do things to quiet the environment where you live or spend time. Double-paned glass doors or windows and carpeting on the floor—or even on the wall—can deaden sound and allow some protection from unwanted sound intrusions. Learn to lower the noise levels in your environment. Tone down the music and turn off the television once in a while. The environment can also be softened with music; overstuffed furniture; simple, pleasant-to-the-eye décor; and harmonious colors.

Anne: I used to watch television to help me shut off my brain. But when I watched the news or a TV program, it seemed to disquiet my mind, and I would go to sleep more agitated. When I moved to Hawaii, I didn't take my TV with me. What I've learned is that TV did not shut off my brain—it gave me more things to think about.

My apartment now is very quiet. Not having TV noise on makes a big difference. I feel more calm and relaxed without TV in my life. It has made all the difference in the world. It's as if the quietness has helped me to find an off button. I'm really at peace here. I feel centered, and I like that.

You can learn to separate yourself periodically from the crowded stimuli you live with. Try putting a "Do Not Disturb" sign on the door. You can make time for quiet activities like browsing the libraries or museums. Or seek the quiet places in the great outdoors. In these ways you can temporarily eliminate noisy, chaotic activities.

Gale: Something that has often helped me is to go to a hot tub or a swimming pool where I float on my back. With my ears just under the water, I hear a roaring sound. The act of floating this way and the white noise that the water creates in my head relaxes and calms me and slows down my thought processes.

But there are good sounds going on in the world, right along with the obnoxious ones. Most of the time, sounds of children playing and laughing can be pleasant. These playful sounds of life can be some of the greatest sounds of all, the sounds of living.

The perception of touch is also affected by stimulus augmentation. Letting people know to what extent you are comfortable being touched is important. It is also important to be comfortable physically with the right shoes and clothes.

Robin: Something that has helped me a lot with my stimulus augmentation is wearing comfortable clothing. When I have on tight or poor-fitting clothes, my stress levels go way up. It's not something most people think of when we talk about changing our environment. But it does make a difference.

Touching

Touching in not just pleasurable; it is a human need. As we have tended to become isolated as a society—distanced as families and neighbors, whether because of the increased use of technology, the impersonal workplace, or our fear of crime and abuse—physical contact has suffered. The skin needs nurturing.

Skin is the body's largest organ and often the most neglected. Be good to your skin by wearing soft clothing made of natural fabrics that breathe. Protect it from sun damage. Use moisturizers to protect it from dryness. Touching is a great source of pleasure. Blood pressure can be lowered by petting a furry animal (especially one like Sammy). A hug can be very therapeutic. "Healing touch" is not just a phrase; it is an experience.

Enjoying Water

There is a natural healing power to water. We use water for hydration, cleansing, nutrition, relaxation, and recreation. It stimulates, warms, cools, soothes, and fulfills the need for touch.

Showering does more than cleanse. Use it to experience the healing power of water. Try standing under a shower and enjoying the feel of the water on your skin. To awaken your senses and increase circulation, alternate hot and cold water. Try a shower massager, or shower at night with only a night light and imagine that you are standing in a waterfall.

Like a shower, a bath can also be used for more than cleansing. In the bath, water can touch you all over, can embrace you. It can soothe and relax you through its buoyancy, warmth, and gentleness. A hot tub provides much the same luxurious pleasure. In addition, its whirlpool jets can relieve an aching, sore body as well as soothe and relax muscles.

Swimming is one of few activities by which we can get complete exercise and a sensuous experience at the same time. Lap swimming can be meditative as well. If you wear goggles and earplugs, the sound of water gurgling as you swim contributes to the relaxation. Because the water supports every part of the body, this form of exercise can seem effortless. The water supports as it caresses.

It is not necessary to know how to swim to enjoy a dip in a pool. You can do water exercise or just splash and have fun. The weightless feeling is very pleasurable when you can let go and just be. Enjoy the buoyancy of the water by submerging yourself and floating to the top. There is nothing quite as luxurious as surrendering to the water by floating on your back, arms to your sides, eyes closed, and the water supporting you. Relax and feel the water surround you.

Music

Some sounds soothe and some invigorate. The sounds of music, waterfalls, rustling leaves, ocean waves, or birds singing are usually pleasing and enjoyable. Other sounds are pleasing to some people and not to other people. Be selective and choose sounds that help you feel more comfortable. Careful choice of music or sound can enhance the pleasure of daily life. It can brighten spirits or calm them down, depending on the type of music played.

Music is powerful. Music that is paced at fifty beats per minute is calming and relaxing. It can also provide a quiet background for study. Music energizes the body through vibration. Singing or humming is stress relieving. Music sets the stage for the body to be in balance and thereby supports the healing process.

David: A memorable magic moment occurred for me as I was going through a car wash. A Kenny G CD was on, and as I glided through the suds, I was cleansed by the sounds of the music; just rub-a-dub-dubbing along through the car wash, that sax and I were one. All around the car, music angels were flitting on swooshing wings delivering their rhythmic embrace, fusing me and settling an always fragile equilibrium with soothing resonance and artful elegance. I felt cleaner than the car, my sparkle enhanced by music's medicine.

Music, art, and nature can be especially enjoyable for people with stimulus augmentation. Individuals with the ability to see and hear so much at one time often have an appreciation of details that simply pass others by. When listening to music they hear and experience every instrument. When looking at a painting they are aware of nuances of color not perceived by those less aware. When walking by the ocean they are aware of the sand beneath their feet, the color of the sky, the sound of the seagull, and the grace of the pelican. They notice the size and shape of the shells, the roar of the sea, the regularity of the waves, and the great expanse of the water. And so they have the capacity to experience ecstasy and awe in a way that is unknown to those who can experience only one thing at a time.

CHAPTER 13

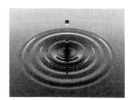

Stress-Reducing Attitudes

WHILE SEARCHING FOR WAYS TO CHANGE your physiology and biochemistry to increase your comfort in sobriety, don't forget that how you feel is also determined by your thoughts, feelings, perceptions, perspectives, and beliefs. You are not a victim of your physiology. You are not powerless over your thoughts, feelings, and attitudes. You can choose how you look at yourself, other people, and the world. In doing so, you can improve your ability to handle stress and the challenges of recovery.

Anxiety Can Be an Opportunity

Anxiety is not necessarily bad. It can call your attention to a need for change, or it can make you mindful of something you've been unaware of. A crisis can be an opportunity.

The question is: Are you going to listen to what the anxiety is telling you or run from it? For many of us, anxiety triggers a desire to consume a substance that relieves anxiety by releasing endorphins that help us relax. When this has been our way of reducing anxiety and we choose not to use that method anymore, we need other ways to decrease anxiety. If we don't find them, our level of anxiety continues to escalate.

You may believe that discomfort is proof that you are doing something wrong. Discomfort does not always mean that there is a problem. It may mean that something wonderful is about to happen. But to get to the other side of anxiety it is necessary to experience it and not try to make it go away. If you face it, it can help you discover what you believe about your situation, yourself, and your life. Pain can motivate you to move toward your dreams. But if your goal is to make it go away, you can usually find a way to do that—temporarily. If you can handle the discomfort without looking for pain control, then you may find yourself looking at a new opportunity.

Don't let anxiety get you off the track from where you want to go, whether your goal is staying sober or changing your career. Don't let fear block your dreams. The faith and courage you need to follow your dreams comes from the inner wisdom that knows what you need to do. When you listen to the voice that encourages you to go ahead, one step at a time, the anxiety lessens, and you can walk into opportunities you thought would always remain just dreams. Change demands risk, but change is an exciting part of life. Taking the risk to try something new keeps life exciting and full of surprises.

It May Be in Your Perception

Sometimes anxiety is due to what we perceive is going on, rather than what is actually going on. We interpret events according to our perceptions. If we expect to be rejected, we may perceive that we have been, when in fact we haven't been. If we believe ourselves incapable of doing a good job, we may think we are doing a poor job, when in fact we are doing well.

But anxiety does not always mean that something is wrong with your thinking; sometimes it means something is wrong with someone else's thinking. You can experience anxiety because others do not recognize or support your worth. In such situations, you might choose to avoid a crisis by accepting the other person's belief, but you experience anxiety when you settle for less than you deserve or are capable of.

There is a difference between feeling bad and being bad; the difference between fact and feelings. It is important to identify what your feelings are, respect them, and learn to express them in appropriate ways; but it is also important to recognize that these feelings may be based on inaccuracies. Sometimes, instead of changing our situation, we need to change our perception of it. In order to do that, it is necessary to tolerate discomfort long enough to figure out what the facts really are and what action is appropriate.

Learning to look at a situation differently can increase serenity even when there is nothing you can do to change it. Step back and refocus. Evaluate whether something is worth fighting for or about. Not every argument is worth trying to win. Set yourself free from the anxiety of unrealistic expectations.

Believe You Can Change

When we are unaware of effective ways to bring about change, we often apply the same would-be cures over and over again more intensely, more diligently. The more ineffective our actions, the harder we try, despite growing despair. If you are trying to pound a nail with a marshmallow, it doesn't help to hit harder. As you come to believe that nothing can be solved, you lose hope of anything getting better. A common statement that shuts out the possibility of change is "That's just the way I am." This is a way of saying, "Don't expect anything different from me. I will always be like I am."

Believing you can achieve something empowers you. This is not just the power of positive thinking. If you believe something is possible, you will invest more energy in making it happen than if you really don't believe it can happen. You have more energy to invest. Hope is energizing. It re-inspires confidence; it fires imagination and creativity. You do have choices, even when you don't know what they are. Feeling powerless is not the same as being powerless.

There are some payoffs in being powerless to change. Some of us get nurturing from being helpless; most of us do to some extent. Painful situations allow us to nurture ourselves in certain ways because we deserve it. After all, look at what we have suffered. We may believe we would have to give up nurturing ourselves if it was no longer a reward for our suffering.

Are people with an addiction victims? Well, in a sense, yes: victims of physiology. You didn't choose your body. If you were born that way, it certainly isn't your fault, and even those things you've done to contribute to the problem you did in the sincere attempt to make things better. People with addictions are also victims of public opinion and prejudice, but because this condition is not your fault does not mean you are not responsible for the choices you make as a result. It may be that heredity, your environment, and society have contributed to your situation. But, regardless of the contributing factors, you are the one that has to do something about it.

You can change. People change all the time. Change is a part of life. Believing you can do something not only gives you hope, it increases your chances for success. If you go to the gym and work out, you are not creating new muscles; you are just making the ones you already have stronger. The same is true for the abilities you need to change. You already have them. You just need to strengthen them. The most essential ingredient in the ability to change is courage. Courage is not lack of fear. It is taking action despite fear. It is being willing to risk failure or exposure. Many people are so immobilized by fear of failure that they live timid, cautious lives. They cannot act because they are so afraid of what will happen if they fail. If you want to develop courage, give yourself permission to fail. Courage gives you the freedom to try.

Accept Your Limitations

But believing you can change is not a magic answer. There are some things you can't change. You probably can't change the way your body responds to mood-altering substances when you ingest them. You probably can't change the way you metabolize alcohol when you drink. You can't change yourself into a 6 foot, 5 inch person if you are at your adult height of 5 feet, 4 inches. There are some things that just *are*. When you can't accept some things as they are, you are always going to be frustrated. You will expend energy on things you have no power over, neglecting things you do have the power to change.

Anxiety can occur when you do not accept your limitations, when you fail to acknowledge that there are some problems you can't solve. The limitations that reality puts on us can be stressful. We cannot always be perfect. We cannot always be the best.

Mistakes are not failure. They're just mistakes. A mistake is not failure unless you refuse to learn from it. If you look at a mistake as an opportunity to learn rather than as failure, it can just be a step in your success. Most of us learn as much from what we do wrong as from what we do right. We learn what works and what doesn't work. We learn what to do differently the next time. Seeing mistakes as steps in the learning process allows us to use them as assets.

Applying the Serenity Prayer

Wisdom for recovery lies in the words of the Serenity Prayer:

God grant me the serenity to accept the things I cannot change, courage to change things I can, and wisdom to know the difference.

Before you develop the serenity of acceptance or the courage to change, it is necessary to learn to tell the difference.

Learning about addiction and recovery will help you make responsible choices in relation to your condition. Numerous mistaken beliefs about addiction can lead to trying to change what you are powerless over. When you learn that chronic abstinence symptoms can be reduced by reducing stress, you can take action to change some stressful situations in life. The more you learn about addiction the better able you will be to make responsible choices.

With the process of recovery, there is the growing realization that the freedom to choose comes with continued sobriety. You are free to change your own behavior; mind-altering chemicals are no longer making your choices. With the freedom to choose comes responsibility. You are free to make responsible choices.

You will find some things standing in the way of responsible behavior. But changing means taking risks. It takes courage to risk. It takes courage to change. You may make some mistakes along the way, but that's how you learn what works and what doesn't.

We create our own serenity by our attitudes and our spiritual resources. Serenity is a choice. You can fret about what you do not have the power to change—your heredity, the weather, what is in the past, what isn't here yet, other people. Or you can accept those things and reinvest that energy in what you do have the power to control. Serenity is accepting what is and setting yourself free—joyfully—to experience the gift of life and the pleasures of sobriety.

Serenity does not mean you don't have any unpleasant feelings. It means you accept life as it is and do not expend excessive energy fighting against what you are powerless over. It does not mean that you do not get angry or afraid. Serenity means accepting and acknowledging all of your feelings. It is knowing that if you get angry you can handle it without hurting yourself or others. You can be serene and still be sad when your dog dies. Serenity is acceptance that your feelings are valid so you don't have to be ashamed or feel guilty about them.

Serenity is also knowing that what you feel and what you do about your feelings are not the same thing. You can be afraid and not run from what you are afraid of. You can be angry and not become violent. You can be sad and not give up on life. You can learn ways to express your feelings that are appropriate and healing.

Perhaps the real secret of serenity is in living in the present—being present in the moment. There is little serenity in replaying what has already happened or waiting for some time in the future to enjoy life. If you are living for tomorrow you are missing out on today. Serenity increases as the experience of being present and comfortable in the moment increases.

"One day at a time" is a slogan learned in AA that is helpful in recovery because it teaches one to focus on the present. Sometimes it can be broken down to one moment at a time. Now is all you have. The past is gone. You cannot change it. The future is not here yet. You cannot experience it. The present is where life is lived. Trying to live in the past or future robs you of the only life you have—the present.

CHAPTER 14

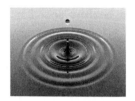

Enriching Life

WE ALL HAVE A NEED FOR HARMONY IN OUR LIVES; balancing our lives is living so that all parts are in harmony. While struggling with addiction your life may have become chaotic and unpredictable. At times you may have felt the insecurity of living on the edge—the edge of despair, the edge of giving up, the edge of complete loss of control. You may have felt the impact physically, mentally, emotionally, socially, and spiritually. You may have been out of harmony with yourself, others, and the world.

When we are focused on drinking or not drinking, we are out of balance, trying to do the impossible. Like a top that can't spin when it is not evenly weighted, we are drained of energy by our efforts to keep an unbalanced life in motion. When we are not getting as much energy from life as it drains from us, we are out of balance.

Balance creates energy; as we grow in recovery, we revitalize and rebalance all areas of our lives. We are released from attempting to achieve unattainable goals. Sickness and disharmony are replaced with wholeness and balance. We are revitalized, reconnected with healthy living. When we are living a balanced life, we are living responsibly, with time for family, job, friends, and ourselves. Balanced living includes attention to health care with proper focus on nutrition, exercise, and rest; attention to personal growth with proper regard to attitudes, feelings, and actions; a healthy social network; and enriching spiritual life.

At first, recovery may seem chaotic. So much focus and attention on self-care may seem to put your life even more out of balance. It may seem that you are adding to an already-too-full schedule of activities, causing you to neglect other things that are important. But you cannot integrate good self-care into a balanced life until you learn the basic how-to's. Unavoidably, even in a life that is well balanced, special needs will arise and will cause you to focus on one aspect of living to the temporary exclusion of others. Beginning recovery is such a time. Learning good self-care habits and putting them into practice take time and energy, it's true, but after a while these practices become a predictable part of life.

As recovery becomes normal, you can move beyond basic self-care requirements—eating routines, exercise plans, and meetings. You can expand recovery. You will come to know yourself better while you become aware of the balance between too much and too little, responsibility to yourself and to others, time for work and time for play, time for activity and time for rest.

Balance of Body, Mind, and Spirit

We cannot look to any one aspect of life for all the answers. Because we are composed of many parts, we derive strength from many sources. Balanced living means we are healthy physically and psychologically and have healthy relationships. We recognize that each part of our lives impacts the others. We are no longer focused on only one aspect of life. We strive for and are motivated toward wholesome living.

Physical health allows psychological growth: When we feel good, we find it is easier to think about our attitudes and values and to work on eliminating shame, guilt, and anger. Psychological health allows us to do more easily those things that keep our bodies well. Healthy relationships support our personal growth.

But the whole is more than the sum of the parts. There is something more that is part of a whole person. Let's call it spirit. The spirit is more than just another part. It includes body, mind, feelings, behavior, and relationships, and it joins them all into a whole. The parts cannot be healthy until the whole is.

Balance Between Work and Play

Life is learning, and we learn better when we are having fun. For too many of us, fun is what we do when all the serious stuff (work) is done. Thinking this way keeps us imprisoned in the belief that we can live only on the weekends, on vacation, in retirement, or when we win the lottery.

Children do not make a distinction between work and play, they just experience life. Most adults have lost that ability. To the extent that we can recapture it, we allow ourselves to enjoy whatever we are doing, whatever we call it. Of course, we can't eliminate all activities that we do not especially enjoy; some tasks will resist being transformed from travail into treat. That is part of life. But it is still possible to enjoy a sense of accomplishment for doing them and to appreciate what we learn from the experience—and equally important to give ourselves opportunity for the activities we do enjoy.

Balance Between Relaxation and Stimulation

Sometimes an unbalanced life means we need to learn to take life easier; sometimes it means we need more activities that stimulate and invigorate us. Rest is not doing nothing; it is enjoying the freedom to do anything.

We can be reenergized through both activity and inactivity. Research indicates that we need a balance of brain chemicals that stimulate us and those that calm us down. Some people prefer activities that produce upper chemistry; others tend to go for a downer chemistry. Both types of activity do promote feelings of well-being. But while all of us have our preference, most of us need some mixture of both types in order to live harmoniously with ourselves.

In recovery we may need to find new ways to feel calm or stimulated. Watching television or reading are good calming activities, but relaxation usually needs to be balanced by some activities that are physically stimulating (such as dancing) or mentally stimulating (playing a game or engaging in meaningful conversation). Relaxing means more than putting our feet up, although it certainly includes giving ourselves permission to do that. It also means getting our feet moving.

The balance of inactivity and activity also produces a balance of certain types of brainwaves. When we are active, especially mentally active, we usually produce beta brainwaves. When we are more mentally relaxed, we experience alpha and theta waves. Deep concentration produces a beta state; relaxation exercises produce an alpha or theta state. All mental states are essential to our total well-being, spending an inordinate amount of time in any one creates an imbalance. We create balance with variety in our activities.

Balance Between Giving and Receiving

For many of us, the most difficult aspect of our lives to balance is fulfilling our responsibility to ourselves and our responsibility to others. Placing care of ourselves high on our list of priorities does not mean we do not also care for other people. Nor does giving to other people, even sacrificing for them, mean we should neglect our own recovery or our own growth. When we love ourselves, we take care of ourselves. When we love others, we allow them to take responsibility for their own lives as much as possible—but we support their growth, in whatever ways we can, without damaging ourselves.

As with other areas of recovery, our ability to provide for our own needs while responding to the needs of others expands as our recovery skills increase. At first, we may need to concentrate on our own needs as we learn to implement components of a self-care program. As those activities become a normal part of life, we are able to become more involved in supporting someone else. Paradoxically, giving often comes back to us as a gift.

As her recovery expanded, Marilyn found that giving to others benefited her own growth. She put up in her car a little sign that read "Pass It On," and often took people who did not have transportation to the doctor, or the grocery store, or to AA meetings. She found time to listen when others needed someone to talk to. When anyone asked her what they could do to repay her, she said, "Pass it on." Recently while a friend was in her home, Marilyn mentioned that she was unable to repaint her woodwork because she was allergic to the paint fumes. The friend said, "I'll paint your woodwork while you are on vacation and will air out your house before you get back." Marilyn was deeply touched that someone would offer to do that for her. The friend, seeing Marilyn's reaction, said, "I'm just passing it on."

When we pass it on, we build a sense of community. When we just repay what has been done for us, we only balance the scales. The world is a better place to be when we are passing it on. A new energy is created that keeps on giving.

We need other people; our growth is dependent upon them. At the same time, we need to give to other people. We need to be concerned about others and contribute to their well-being. Through interaction with others we give and receive the feedback necessary for continuing growth. We cannot grow in a vacuum.

Many of us have not been able to achieve the balance of giving and receiving because we do not know how to love ourselves. Those of us who have lived in shame, who have felt defective and unacceptable, may feel unworthy of love and acceptance from others or from ourselves. When our recovery enables us to accept ourselves as we are, we are better able to have mutually supportive relationships with others.

We need strong social networks to nurture us and provide a sense of belonging. We need reciprocal relationships in which we feel valued as we value others, and experience the satisfaction of giving and receiving.

Spiritual Balance

Spiritual balance means we are in harmony with ourselves, with our values, with others, and with God. Step eleven of AA gives us guidance for achieving spiritual balance:

> Sought through prayer and meditation to improve our conscious contact with God as we understood him, praying only for knowledge of His will for us and the power to carry that out.

Just as we don't have to have any special concept of God to do this, neither do we have to use any certain definition of prayer or meditation.

But this step is not about trying to get our higher power to do what we want. It is about aligning our will with a higher will. It is about getting in touch with a power that will help us increase our understanding, our knowledge, our courage, and our willingness to live wholesome lives.

Prayer does not change God, but changes him who prays.

Søren Kierkegaard

Spiritual wholeness is living in harmony with what we believe and value. Shame and guilt result from lack of harmony between our values and our behavior. Conscious contact with a higher power, increased knowledge of that power's will for us, and the power to carry that out enable us to find harmony between what we believe and what we do. We are thus freed from the burden of guilt and shame to find spiritual fulfillment.

Living in balance does not mean we do not have bad days. We still have our ups and downs; we still experience sadness, anger, fatigue, disappointment. We accept these feelings when they are appropriate. We don't have to be ashamed of them or feel guilty for having them. We allow ourselves to experience a whole range of feelings, but we don't let them control us. And we know how to take action that will prevent these emotions from triggering regression. A wholesome, harmonious life does not mean we never do things we regret or feel bad about. It means that we don't need to become discouraged by our inability to be perfect.

When we are living in balance, we accept our humanness

and strive for progress. We seek to eliminate activities that cause us to go to extremes at the expense of other important parts of life. We give up the need for immediate gratification in order to achieve a lifestyle that is more fulfilling and meaningful. Harmony in all aspects of life allows us the balance to go beyond the struggle of using drugs, and to enter into the experience of joyful living.

Joyful Living

Is there a voice within you, calling you to dream and to believe in your dreams? Listen to that voice. It is your creative spirit. It is calling you to live fully and passionately, to risk and to play. It is calling you to joy. As you listen to that voice and respond to it, it will become stronger. It is calling you to see yourself as a person of integrity and worth, one who has unique dreams and unique talents to offer the world. Responding to that special call leads us on a journey that goes beyond preventing relapse, beyond just getting back to ground zero. Seeing the possibilities of life and seeing ourselves with the potential for attaining wholeness gives purpose and meaning to our journey. That sense of purpose and meaning is a result and a facilitator of healing.

Replacing self-defeating lifestyles with hope and meaning takes self-care beyond maintenance into abundant living. Abundant living means more than material abundance. It means lives that are rich physically, mentally, socially, and spiritually. Moving beyond the issues of using or not using, we replace artificial ways of feeling good with natural ways. The brain creates positive chemistry and generates positive thoughts and feelings, leading to an expectation of opportunities and new possibilities. Life becomes an adventure.

We do not become aware of the possibilities for abundance

if our main interest in life is the prevention of relapse. If we don't see something bright and new to move into, we can only long for what we are giving up. If we focus on an abundant life, and stay focused on it, then we will hope for that abundance, expect it, and seek it. If we feed our hopes, our fears will starve to death.

People who don't know how to live fully use temporary, artificial substitutes for the real riches life offers. But we know that in the long run these substitutes only increase pain, deadening senses rather than awakening them.

People who have used addictive living to produce pleasure or relieve pain, and who don't know any other way to feel good or to relieve their pain, will eventually go back to addictive use. If our emphasis is on not drinking, then we're focused on what we are not doing; we're saying no to life. It is time we say yes—yes to living fully and joyfully.

A Spiritual Awakening

Step twelve of AA says:

> Having had a spiritual awakening as a result of these steps, we tried to carry this message to others and to practice these principles in all our affairs.

A spiritual awakening occurs as we go beyond the struggle of controlling our addiction and, having found meaning beyond ourselves, we discover the joys of living. We experience enriching pleasures that take us beyond just not using. We actively participate in life rather than passively hoping life will offer us something good along the way.

A spiritual awakening occurs as we learn that spirituality is not separate from our daily lives, but encompasses life and brings new meaning to all our affairs. Although spirituality must be defined by each of us for ourselves alone, it is interesting to note that Webster's dictionary tells us the word is derived from *spiritus*, which means "of breathing" and "an animating or vital principle held to give life." Our spiritual awakening allows this animating force to be breathed into all areas of our existence.

Spirituality and religion is not the same thing. Religion is a set of beliefs about the spiritual and the practices based on those beliefs. Religion certainly is a means by which some people connect to the spiritual, but we may experience a spiritual awakening without being affiliated with a specific religion or religious denomination. A spiritual awakening is a personal experience that opens the door to meaningful and creative living.

Living Creatively

When creativity is blocked, the result is powerlessness and impotence. To live creatively is to give expression to our inner selves. A creative spirit calls us to create laughter, love, forgiveness, and healing in ourselves and others. Creativity may be expressed through cooking, gardening, caring for children, caring for elderly, writing, playing, making love, decorating, painting, dancing, journaling, teaching, counseling, repairing, designing and so on.

The call to creativity is a call to joy, zest, and a sense of meaning and purpose. Are you listening to that call? Failure to experience life's meaningful pleasures creates a void that is often filled with destructive pleasures. They offer no hope and no joy.

We need to sharpen our senses rather than deaden them. We need to wake up and see what is already around us. Someone has said boredom comes from lack of involvement. Get involved. Celebrate life. Celebrate people and animals and all creation. Celebrate yourself.

We must learn to reawaken and keep ourselves awake, not by mechanical aids, but by an infinite expectation of the dawn, which does not forsake us in our soundest sleep.

Henry David Thoreau

To live creatively and joyfully does not mean being happy all the time. Struggle is a normal and usually necessary part of creativity, just as labor is a normal part of giving birth. To live creatively is to experience a fullness of life; it is to be open to suffering as well as to pleasure. Pain is woven into life's pleasures and comforts, and is even essential to them. When we turn away from struggle, we turn away from progress, and a deeper pain grows. To escape from normal pain and struggle is to escape from life.

Compassion

Our pain can never be erased without compassion—"an awakening of passion with all creation."[1] Compassionate living means maintaining creative relationships with the earth, the creatures of the earth, and other people. The reason we damage the earth, one another, and ourselves is that we are out of harmony. Harmony results from valuing all creation, including ourselves—our bodies, minds, and spirits. Destructiveness comes from not honoring life. Compassion is reverence for life, including a reverence for our own specialness and our own beauty.

The most beautiful experience we can have is the mysterious. It is the fundamental emotion which stands at the cradle of true art and true science. Whoever does not know it and can no longer wonder, no longer marvel, is as good as dead.

Albert Einstein

Compassion brings responsibility, not out of duty, but out of our wanting to care for what we cherish and value. What do you cherish? What are you enthusiastic about? The word *enthusiasm* means "spirit." Do you have life-spirit? Do you have self-spirit? Compassion is a call to courage. Discouragement kills faith and hope and spirit. Courage awakens and empowers. It empowers us to walk into our dreams with hope and enthusiasm.

An important aspect of recovery is giving to others out of compassion and concern. Our own wounds become a resource for healing: Out of our suffering come the wisdom and understanding to pass the healing on. Those of us for whom addiction has been the object and focus of life have the opportunity to give to others in recovery. Having lived through much anguish, we are survivors of a condition that has eaten the very center out of our self-esteem. Out of this struggle, we gain insight and compassion to give to and receive from others. Sharing these principles with others is important in keeping them active in our own lives.

Nothing renews commitment like sharing the joy that results from the commitment . . . sharing keeps the light on and the spirit high.

Larrene Hagaman[2]

Sharing with others keeps the growth process going. Without it, we retreat back into ourselves and allow the old shames to creep in and take over. Carrying the message allows life to take on an "other" focus rather than just a "self" focus. As we give to others, we reflect their worth and see our own worth reflected in them. This sense of unity creates a deeper sense of the interconnectedness we have with others and with all living things.

Freedom

Freedom of choice is the greatest opportunity we have. We can choose life; we can choose to take a different path no matter where we have been. We can choose to use the resources we have to become what we were created to be. Or we can choose to hang on to feelings of inadequacy that keep us locked into discouragement.

As we become aware of our ability to use our own judgment and, through that exercise, to assert more control over our own lives, we begin to see our potential instead of our shortcomings. We stop seeing other people through defensive eyes as we learn to see them in the light of our empowering interaction with them. We see that we, as individuals working and playing together, can become more than we could in isolation.

We really do not grow or gain in self-esteem by adhering to the wisdom of the self alone. We need, ultimately, to feel a sense of belonging. We need to be involved with others, to exchange perceptions with them, to give and get support. We need others to help us stop the inner war that is fueled by shame and distorted pictures of ourselves.

Freedom comes from an emphasis on what we are seeking rather than on what we are avoiding. If emphasis is on the not (what we are not consuming, what habits we are not engaging in), then we are always aware of what is lacking in our lives. Life seems to mean deprivation and restriction. But as we move into replacement activities our picture of life changes: We see and we expect abundance. Armed as never before against regression, we are freed to spiral up into new aspects of growth.

Serendipity

A bonus on the recovery journey, serendipity is the good fortune of discovering something good while seeking something else. It happens when we compare what we have been seeking with what we have found, and decide that the thing we've found is even better than that which we'd sought. Many people, out of their pain and acceptance, have experiences in which their insights and benefits far surpass their expectations of merely staying on track.

The person at an AA meeting who says "I'm a grateful alcoholic" is describing this experience of serendipity. She has found on her healing journey much more than she ever expected, more than only maintaining abstinence, more than just hanging on. A new way of life has opened up for her. Expecting serendipity means living in a way that says, "Today I can experience only the present. As I do, I expect the unexpected. I have a choice to truly experience today, as fully as I can."

A certain story has held particular meaning for us, and we wish to share it with you. We hope it will help light the path that you take in recovery.

There was once a young farm boy whose father was away and whose mother asked him to go to the barn in the dark to feed the animals. But he was afraid of the dark. His mother assured him that the lantern would furnish the light he needed to get there and back. "But the lantern only shines its light a short way in front of me," he said. "I can't see all the way to the barn." Then, handing him the lantern, his mother took him outside. "Now, son," she said, "just take one step toward the barn." As he took one step the light moved ahead of him. "All you have to do," his mother told him, "is take one step at a time and the light will go before you all the way."

There is a light that goes ahead of us on our recovery journey. We can see as far as we need to see to live a full and joyful life. We don't have to wait until we get to the end of the journey to begin living or to experience the light. As you take your next steps into recovery, watch for the light that illuminates your path.

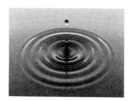

Putting It All Together

Bridging the Gaps
Winchester, Virginia

Stanley Stokes, MS, LPC, CCDC, established Bridging the Gaps to bridge the gaps between what is commonly done in treatment and what is possible with biochemical rebalancing. This process of rebalancing brain chemistry is a model in progress at BTG. This includes determining individual needs and providing the appropriate nutrients and treatments that will allow readjustment of the body's own physiology and the natural components necessary for a quality life in recovery.

To help rapidly reverse biochemical deficiencies and imbalances and chronic abstinence symptoms, Bridging the Gaps offers intravenous and oral nutritional therapy for residential clients, alumni clients, and outpatients.

In addition, BTG programs incorporate many types of treatment, including acu-detox, nutritional counseling, physical exercise, massage, Reiki, yoga, and others to help in people's recovery. All programs are enhanced with a relapse prevention skills training program developed by Merlene and David Miller.

By adhering to a program of healthy eating habits, structured daily exercise, meditation, relaxation, and restful sleep, the recovering individual will be much better equipped to stay sober. Having rebalanced brain chemistry and identified warning signs, triggers, and high-risk situations in a real-life setting and actively participated in a twelve-step program, the recovering resident can enjoy the encouragement and support needed to make the transition to sober living.

The intravenous therapy at Bridging the Gaps includes six to ten days of nutrients delivered in four-hour periods by a nurse practitioner supervised by a medical doctor. For patients who have received intravenous and oral nutritional therapy along with the other treatments offered, Bridging the Gaps claims a 90 percent recovery rate over a twelve-month period. (www.bridgingthegaps.com)

Community Addiction Recovery Association
Sacramento, California

CARA is a nonprofit organization treating chemical dependency with acupuncture, herbal tea, yoga, nutritional supplements, nutrition education, Chinese exercise routines (tai chi and qi gong), and Emotional Freedom Technique, a method of relieving post-traumatic stress and other emotionally charged memories through verbalization of the problem coupled with acupressure. Staff includes licensed acupuncturists and certified practitioners of clinical nutrition and the various mind-body integration techniques offered.

Exercise allows recovering individuals to be reintroduced to their bodies and in the process learn a simple method of stress reduction. The gentle, flowing exercise called tai chi is easy for pregnant or obese women. Qi gong teaches power over breath and body for self-mastery and healing. Yoga integrates mind and body through control of breath, mind, and body. These forms of self-healing are physically satisfying even to those who aren't ready for or are resisting talk therapy.

CARA contracts with individual treatment facilities to provide any or all of these services on site. Future plans include a newsletter and educational materials introducing both acupuncture and targeted nutrition to the recovery community. (www.carasac.org)

Counseling and Mediation Services
Wichita, Kansas

Carol Cummings, MSW, an addiction counselor in private practice as part of Counseling and Mediation Services, uses a variety of alternative treatment methods in an outpatient setting. First, the client is assessed, usually by a psychiatrist, to evaluate any serotonin or dopamine deficiencies or other neurochemical imbalances. Appropriate amino acid supplements and vitamins are then recommended. Clients are introduced to a variety of stress-reducing techniques, including deep breathing, progressive relaxation, meditation, prayer, music, and art.

Aromatherapy is used to help reduce stress and promote wellness. Classical music, especially Mozart, works directly on the brain for relaxation, healing, learning, and enhancing creativity.

Cummings incorporates a variety of bilateral stimulation exercises to help reduce trauma and enhance healing of the brain. She teaches an exercise routine to be used every morning that's designed to increase oxygen flow to the brain and increase and balance electrical energy to the neocortex. This allows choice by providing access to reason rather than reaction and increases polarity across cell membranes for more efficient thought processing and focused attention. (www.counselingandmeditation.org)

Excel Treatment
Denver, Colorado

Excel is an outpatient addiction treatment program with a treatment philosophy based on research that shows that the cause and treatment for addiction centers on the brain—not just the mind. Treatment at Excel features intravenous and oral amino acids, vitamins, and minerals to help reverse genetic and drug-related damage, thereby boosting the brain's ability to absorb dopamine. The intravenous therapy is administered under the supervision of a licensed physician for about ten days. It is administered as a painless drip over three to four hours for ten treatments and is followed by weekly group counseling for six months. Along with the IV program, which has consistently produced dramatic results in reversing physiological addictions, Excel also includes a comprehensive psychological counseling program that supports the continuation of a new lifestyle important to long-term success.

Excel claims a greater than 80 percent success rate over a period of twelve months. Dr. Thomas Levy, medical director of Excel, says, "We have now been administering the IV treatment for all types of addictive behavior with incredible success." He reports that patients experience no cravings and no withdrawal symptoms. Tamea Sisco adds that safety is important, so all amino acids used are FDA-approved. In addition to psychological counseling, other modalities such as acupuncture, massage, and ionic foot baths are used to enhance the effectiveness of treatment at Excel. (www.exceltreatment.com)

ExecuCare Addiction Recovery Center
Norcross, Georgia

ExecuCare ARC is an outpatient treatment program that utilizes an intravenous formulation of amino acids, minerals, and vitamins for neurotransmitter restoration (NTR), developed by Dr. William Hitt of the Hitt Clinic in Tijuana, Mexico. The formulation is administered over a ten-day period by a registered nurse under a doctor's supervision.

NTR treats the physical aspects of the disease of addiction by restoring normal brain functioning. ExecuCare recognizes that counseling is a key component that impacts behavior and has arranged for counseling to be available to clients after they leave the ExecuCare Program. (www.execucarearc.com)

Inner Balance Health Center
Loveland, Colorado

Inner Balance Health is a residential alcohol and drug treatment center that has been helping people with alcohol and drug addictions since 1998. Inner Balance uses a combination of biochemical restoration with natural supplements (not medications), bioelectrical stimulation, an exercise program, yoga, meditation, personalized nutritional planning and counseling, talk therapy, addiction education, and lifestyle coaching—resulting in a successful sobriety in over 80 percent of its clients. (www.innerbalancehealthcenter.com)

LifeStream Nutritional Consultation and Products
Prescott, Arizona

This is a consulting program based on the experience and scientific research of Dr. Charles Gant, MD, PhD, NMD. The service is based on the premise that substance abuse problems are the result of biochemical imbalances that disrupt the normal workings of brain cells. Information is gathered through a questionnaire process or with personal assessment by Dr. Gant or Debra Manka. Products (Dopamine Pak, GABA Pak, Endorphin Pak, or Serotonin Pak) are recommended according to the brain chemistry imbalances indicated. Supplements come in a thirty-day supply of sixty individually wrapped packets. The supplement "paks" are based on the research reported in the book *End Your Addiction Now* by Gant and are made up of the appropriate combination of amino acids, vitamins, and minerals. Using the nutrient paks can help restore neurotransmitter production by supplying the brain with the raw materials needed to rebalance chemistry. (www.lifestream-solutions.com)

LifeStream Solutions and Medaus Pharmacy
Prescott, Arizona

LifeStream Solutions promotes the application of innovative science-based solutions—especially intravenous and oral nutritional therapy—to the problem of chemical dependency. LifeStream is dedicated to providing solutions that not only help people get sober but help people stay sober.

Along with Medaus, LifeStream offers training for medical professionals in the application of intravenous nutritional therapy and for other addiction treatment professionals in the integration of nutritional therapy into traditional treatment.

LifeStream Solutions is affiliated with Medaus Compound Pharmacy to ensure the highest quality nutritional products and ingredients. Medaus is a full-service pharmacy dedicated to the preparation of compounded medications. Compounding is the art of preparing customized medications designed for individual needs. With seventy years of combined compounding experience, the staff has established a reputation among physicians by providing medications and advice that make a difference in the lives of their patients.

Medaus uses only the highest quality active ingredients in every order, prepared to exact specifications, which is why every order filled is 100 percent guaranteed. Medaus ensures a timely response on each order and can assist in obtaining reimbursement from insurance providers.

Together LifeStream and Medaus offer the highest quality and safest ingredients available, affiliation with a network of providers who utilize intravenous nutritional therapy, training in intravenous and oral neuro-nutritional therapy and related therapies, and referral services to providers of intravenous and oral nutritional therapy. (www.lifestream-solutions.com)

Recovery Systems
Mill Valley, California

Julia Ross, MA, is founder and executive director of Recovery Systems, which provides holistic outpatient assessments, counseling, and nutritional therapy, along with medical care for alcohol, drug, and food addictions. Ross is the author of *The Diet Cure* and *The Mood Cure*. The staff of holistic nutritionists, counselors, and physicians is trained by Ross to identify symptoms of neurotransmitter deficiencies and imbalances as well as other nutritional deficiencies and to recommend appropriate treatment for the deficiencies and underlying causes.

Nutritional therapy provides a pro-recovery diet and targeted nutritional supplement protocols. In-office trials of oral amino acids are provided. The initial session is followed by weekly appointments for at least three months (by phone or in person). Oral amino acids—as part of a total nutritional program—are an important part of the treatment recommended to relieve cravings and "false moods." Medical care is provided in the way of examinations, special testing, and prescriptions, as needed. When residential treatment is needed, Recovery Systems personnel work closely with cooperative local facilities.

Intravenous amino acid therapy is available through Recovery Systems when determined advisable, especially for detoxification from mood-altering substances. (www.dietcure.com)

APPENDIX B

CHRONIC ABSTINENCE SYMPTOM SEVERITY SCALE

Circle the number that best indicates the severity of each symptom you are experiencing <u>today</u> (zero indicates the absence of the symptom, 10 represents an extreme intensity level). Answer each question as honestly as possible.

		Low Level									High Level	
1.	Craving/drug or alcohol hunger	0	1	2	3	4	5	6	7	8	9	10
2.	Craving for sweets/sugar/bread	0	1	2	3	4	5	6	7	8	9	10
3.	Loss of appetite	0	1	2	3	4	5	6	7	8	9	10
4.	Overeating/always hungry	0	1	2	3	4	5	6	7	8	9	10
5.	Sense of emptiness/incompleteness	0	1	2	3	4	5	6	7	8	9	10
6.	Anxiety	0	1	2	3	4	5	6	7	8	9	10
7.	Internal shakiness	0	1	2	3	4	5	6	7	8	9	10
8.	Restlessness	0	1	2	3	4	5	6	7	8	9	10
9.	Impulsiveness/act before thinking	0	1	2	3	4	5	6	7	8	9	10
10.	Difficulty concentrating/focusing	0	1	2	3	4	5	6	7	8	9	10
11.	Fuzzy thinking/confusion	0	1	2	3	4	5	6	7	8	9	10
12.	Memory problems	0	1	2	3	4	5	6	7	8	9	10
13.	Depression	0	1	2	3	4	5	6	7	8	9	10
14.	Mood swings	0	1	2	3	4	5	6	7	8	9	10
15.	Negative self-talk	0	1	2	3	4	5	6	7	8	9	10
16.	Irritability/quick tempered	0	1	2	3	4	5	6	7	8	9	10
17.	Impatience	0	1	2	3	4	5	6	7	8	9	10
18.	Daytime sleepiness/drowsiness	0	1	2	3	4	5	6	7	8	9	10
19.	Problems getting to or staying asleep	0	1	2	3	4	5	6	7	8	9	10
20.	Fatigue/lack of energy	0	1	2	3	4	5	6	7	8	9	10
21.	Hypersensitivity to stress	0	1	2	3	4	5	6	7	8	9	10
22.	Hypersensitivity to noise/sight/touch	0	1	2	3	4	5	6	7	8	9	10
23.	Hypersensitivity to pain	0	1	2	3	4	5	6	7	8	9	10
24.	Coordination problems	0	1	2	3	4	5	6	7	8	9	10
25.	Emotional overreaction/numbness	0	1	2	3	4	5	6	7	8	9	10

Total Score Here _____

Use this as your base score and check regularly to see if you are making progress in reducing the severity of chronic abstinence symptoms with brain-healing activities.

Developed by David Miller, Ph.D and James Braly, M.D.

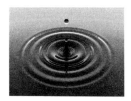

Deficiency Questionnaires

On the following questionnaires, circle the number at the right if you answer "yes" to any of the following questions, then total your points.

SEROTONIN DEFICIENCY QUESTIONNAIRE

Is alcohol your drug of choice?	3
If you have used marijuana, does it have a relaxing effect?	2
Have you ever taken prescription antidepressants, such as Prozac, Paxil, or Zoloft?	5
Have you ever gotten relief from your symptoms by taking 5-HTP or the amino acid tryptophan?	5
Does eating high-sugar foods or processed carbohydrates relax you or relieve your anxiety, or both?	2
Do you often have the sense that you are "out of sync" or not attuned to what's going on around you?	2
Do you have a history of anxious depression — that is, feeling nervous or irritable when you are "down"?	2

Do you have a regular pattern of unexplained rages or
a history of explosive or assaultive behavior?   3
Do you have a history of sleep problems, especially
waking up early and not being able to get back to sleep?   2
Is there a history of depression in your family?   2
Do you often experience symptoms of gastrointestinal
distress, including gas, bloating, loose stools or constipation? 3

Total your circled points _____

Eleven to 14 points means you are probably serotonin-deficient.
Fifteen or more points means you are very probably serotonin-deficient.

CATECHOLAMINE DEFICIENCY QUESTIONNAIRE
(Dopamine and Norepinephrine)

Is either cocaine or amphetamines your drug of choice?   5
Do you smoke cigarettes or use nicotine in another form,
such as smokeless tobacco?
If 1 pack a day or less, 1 point.   1
If 2 packs a day, 2 points.   2
If 3 or more packs, 3 points.   3
Does marijuana excite you or have a "speedy" effect on you?   2
Is there a history of mania in your family?   2
Is there a history of depression in you family?   2
Do you often experience tiredness, loss of energy,
or an inability to feel pleasure?   3
Are you a thrill seeker or risk-taker?   3
Do you respond positively to antidepressant drugs?   5
Do you respond positively to prescription drugs such
as Ritalin, Cylert, Adderall, or amphetamines?   5

Total your circled points _____

Eleven to 14 points means you are probably catecholamine-deficient. Fifteen or more points means you are very probably serotonin-deficient.

ENDORPHIN DEFICIENCY QUESTIONNAIRE

Circle the number at the right if you answer "yes" to any of the following questions, then total your points.

Are heroin, Darvon, codeine, methadone, or other opiates
your drugs of choice?   5

Have you ever had difficulty stopping the use of painkilling
drugs such as codeine, Darvon, methadone or other opiates?   3

Do you use drugs or alcohol to carve out a respite or
"time out" from a very busy, active life?   2

Are you troubled by chronic pain, such as back pain
or headaches?   2

Do you have difficulty enjoying pleasurable experiences
much of the time (and not just when you are feeling down)?   2

Do you have a low pain tolerance?   2

                              Total your circled points_____

Eight to 11 points means you are probably endorphin-deficient. Twelve points or more points means you are very probably endorphin-deficient.

GABA DEFICIENCY QUESTIONNAIRE

Are sedatives or "downers" your drug of choice?   2

Is alcohol your drug of choice?   2

Does alcohol relax you, or help you to sleep?   4

Have you obtained relief from symptoms of anxiety
by taking prescription drugs?   5

Do you often have symptoms such as headache, irritability,
or dizziness when you go four or more hours without food?   5

Do you have a history of panic attacks or severe anxiety?   3

Do you have a tendency to be thin or underweight?   2

Do you have problems sleeping, especially falling asleep?   2

Do you have sugar cravings?   2

Is there a history of anxiety or panic disorder in your family?   2

Total your circled points _____

Eleven to 14 points means you are probably GABA-deficient. Fifteen
or more points means you are very probably GABA-deficient.

Resources

David and Merlene Miller at Miller Associates
800-287-0906
www.miller-associates.org

LifeStream Solutions
www.lifestream-solutions.com

Bridging the Gaps, Inc.
866-711-1234
www.bridgingthegaps.com

Holder Research Institute
800-490-7714 or 305-535-8803

Julia Ross
Recovery Systems
www.dietcure.com

Community Addiction Recovery Association
Sacramento, CA
916-972-1684
www.carasac.org

Excel Treatment
Denver, CO
877-351-5507
www.exceltreatment.com

Carol Cummings at Counseling and Mediation
Wichita, Kansas
316-269-2322

American Massage Therapy Association
www.amtamassage.org

Biofeedback Certification Institute of America
www.bcia.org

Joel Lubar
www.brainwavebiofeedback.com

Notes

Chapter 2

1. For information on the reward system of the brain, see:
   Kenneth Blum and James Payne, *Alcohol and the Addictive Brain.* (New York: The Free Press, 1991).
   G.F. Koob, "Drugs of Abuse: Anatomy, Pharmacology, and Function of Reward Pathways," *Trends in Pharmacological Science* 13 (1992): 177–84.
2. For more information on reward deficiency, see:
   David Comings, et al., "Studies of the Potential Role of the Dopamine D1 Receptor Gene in Addictive Behaviors," *Molecular Psychiatry* 2, No. 1 (1997): 44–56.
   P.M. Conley and R.S. Sparks, "Molecular Genetics of Alcoholism and Other Addictive/Compulsive Disorders," *Alcohol* 16, No. 1 (1998): 85–91.
3. David Miller and Kenneth Blum, *Overload: Attention Deficit Disorder and the Addictive Brain.* (Kansas City, MO: Andrews and McMeel, 1996).
   Ralph Tarter and Kathleen Edwards, "Psychological Factors Associated with the Risk of Alcoholism," *Alcoholism: Clinical and Experimental Research* 12, No. 5 (1988).
4. M.A. Korsten, et al., "High Blood Acetaldehyde Levels After Ethanol Administration: Differences Between Alcoholic and Non-Alcoholic Subjects," *New England Journal of Medicine* 292 (1975): 386–89.
   M.A. Schuckit and V. Rayses, "Ethanol Ingestion: Differences in Blood Acetaldehyde Concentrations in Relatives of Alcoholics and Controls," *Science* 203 (1979): 54–55.
5. V.E. Davis and M.J. Walsh, "Alcohol, Amines, and Alkaloids: A Possible Biochemical Basis for Alcohol Addiction," *Science* 167, No. 920 (1970): 1005–007.

Chapter 3

1. White House Office of National Drug Control Policy, 1996.
2. For more information on these symptoms, see:
   Terence Gorski and Merlene Miller, *Staying Sober: A Guide for Relapse Prevention.* (Independence, MO: Herald House Independence Press, 1986).
3. For more information about Alcoholics Anonymous, see:
   Alcoholics Anonymous. (Alcoholics Anonymous World Services, Inc., 1955)
   Narcotics Anonymous. (C.A.R.E.N.A. Publishing Co., 1982)
4. For more information about the disease model of alcoholism, see:
   I. Maltzman, "Why Alcoholism Is a Disease," *Journal of Psychoactive Drugs* 26 (1994): 13–31.
   James Milam, "The Alcoholism Revolution," *Professional Counselor* 8 (1992).
   Kenneth Blum and James Payne, *Alcohol and the Addictive Brain.* (New York: The Free Press, 1991).
5. *Alcoholics Anonymous.* (Alcoholics Anonymous World Services, Inc., 1955).
6. Katherine Ketcham and William Asbury, *Beyond the Influence.* (New York: Bantam Books, 2000).

Chapter 4

1. Raymond J. Brown, Kenneth Blum, and Michael Trachtenberg, "Neurodynamics of Relapse Prevention: A Neuronutrient Approach to Outpatient DUI Offenders," *Journal of Psychoactive Drugs* 22, No. 2 (April/June 1990).
   G. Kaats, et al., "Effects of Chromium Picolinate Supplementation on Body Composition," *Current Therapeutic Research* 57, No. 10 (1996).
   Kenneth Blum and Michael Trachtenberg, "Neurogenic Deficits Caused by Alcoholism: Restoration by SAAVE," *Journal of Psychoactive Drugs* 20 (1988): 297–312.
   Kenneth Blum, et al., "Neuronutrient Effects on Weight Loss in Carbohydrate Bingers: An Open Clinical Trial," *Current Therapeutic Research* 48 (1990): 217–33.
   Kenneth Blum, et al., "Enkephalinase Inhibition and Precursor Amino Acid Loading Improves Inpatient Treatment of Alcohol and Polydrug Abusers: Double-Blind Placebo-Controlled Study

of the Nutritional Adjunct SAAVE," *Alcohol* 5 (1989): 481–93.

Julia Ross, *The Mood Cure*. (New York: Penguin Group, 2002).

Joan Mathews-Larson, *7 Weeks to Sobriety*. (New York: Fawcett Columbine, rev. ed., 1997).

Charles Gant, *End Your Addiction NOW*. (New York: Warner Books, 2002).

2. Billie Jay Sahley and Katherine M. Birkner, *Heal with Amino Acids and Nutrients*. (San Antonio, TX: Pain and Stress Publications, 2001).

3. Seymour Ehrenpreis, *Degradation of Endogenous Opioids: Its Relevance in Human Pathology and Therapy*. (New York: Raven, 1983).

Arnold Fox, *DLPA to End Chronic Pain and Depression*. (New York: Pocketbooks, 1985).

Seymour Ehrenpreis, "Pharmacology of Enkephalinase Inhibitors: Animal and Human Studies," *Acupuncture Electrotherapy Research* 10, No. 3 (1985): 203–08.

A.E. Anderson, "Lowering Brain Phenylalanine Levels by Giving Other Large Neutral Amino Acids," *Archives of Neurology* 33, No. 10 (1976): 684–86.

K. Budd, "Use of D-phenylalanine, an Enkephalinase Inhibitor, in the Treatment of Intractable Pain," *Advances in Pain Research and Therapy*. J.J. Bonica; J.C. Liebeskind; and D.G. Albe-Fessard, editors. (New York: Raven Press, 1983); 5: 305–08.

G. Donzelle, et al., "Curing Trial of Complicated Oncologic Pain by D-Phenylalanine," *Anesthesia and Analgesia* 38 (1981): 655–58.

Berman A. Fugh and J.M. Cott, Department of Health Care Sciences, George Washington University School of Medicine and Health Sciences, Washington, DC. "Dietary Supplements and Natural Products as Psychotherapeutic Agents," *Psychosomatic Medicine* 61, No. 5 (September 1999): 712–28.

S. Meyers, Lawrence Berkeley National Laboratory, "Use of Neurotransmitter Precursors for Treatment of Depression," *Alternative Medicine Review* 5, No. 1 (February 2000): 64–71.

"PE and Tyrosine in Double Blinded Studies with People Strung Out on Cocaine," *Journal of Psychoactive Drugs* 20, No. 3 (July–September, 1988): 283–95, 315–31, and 333–36.

Yaryura-Tobias, et al., "Phenylalanine for Endogenous

Depression," *Journal of Orthomolecular Psychiatry* 3, No. 2 (1974): 80–81.

4. Eric Braverman, et al., *The Healing Nutrients Within*, (Keats Publishing, Inc. 1997). [Highly recommended. This is the single best reference source on amino acids.]
    S. Meyers, "Use of Neurotransmitter Precursors for Treatment of Depression," *Alternative Medicine Review* 5, No. 1 (February 2000): 64–71.
    C. Benkelfat, et al., "Mood-Lowering Effect of Tryptophan Depletion," *Archives of General Psychiatry* 51 (1994): 687–97.
    W.F. Byerley, et al., "5-Hydroxytryptophan: A Review of Its Anti-Depressant Efficacy and Adverse Effects," *Journal of Clinical Psychopharmacology* 7, No. 3 (1987).
    Farkas, T., et al., "L-Tryptophan in Depression," *Biological Psychiatry* 11, No. 3 (1976).
    E. Hartman and C.L. Spinweber, "Sleep Induced by L-Tryptophan: Effect of Dosages within the Normal Dietary Intake," *Journal of Nervous and Mental Disease* 167, No. 8 (1979).
    S.M. Peuschel, et al., "5-Hydroxytryptophan and Pyridoxine," *American Journal of Diseases of Children* 134 (1980).
    J.E. Reeves and H.W. Laymeyer, "Tryptophan for Insomnia," *Journal of the American Medical Association* 262, No. 19 (November 17, 1989).
    S.L. Satel, et al., "Tryptophan Depletion: An Attenuation of Cue-Induced Cravings for Cocaine," *American Journal of Psychiatry* 152, No. 5 (May 1995).

5. L.E. Banderet; H.R. Lieberman; U.S. Army Research Institute of Environmental Medicine, "Treatment with Tyrosine, a Neurotransmitter Precursor, Reduces Environmental Stress in Humans," *Brain Research Bulletin* 22, No. 4 (April 1989): 759–62.
    J.B. Deijen; J.F. Orlebeke; Department of Psychophysiology, Vrije Universiteit, Amsterdam, The Netherlands, "Effect of Tyrosine on Cognitive Function and Blood Pressure Under Stress," *Brain Research Bulletin* 33, No. 3 (1994): 319–23.
    A.J. Gelenberg and R.J. Wurtman, "L-Tyrosine in Depression," *The Lancet* (October 1980).
    I.K. Goldberg, "L-Tyrosine in Depression," *The Lancet* (August 1980).

H. Lehnert, et al., "Neurochemical and Behavioral Consequences of Acute, Uncontrollable Stress: Effects of Dietary Tyrosine," *Brain Research* 303, No. 2 (June 1984): 215–23.

D.K. Reinstein, et al., "Neurochemical and Behavioral Consequences of Stress: Effect of Dietary Tyrosine," *Journal of the American College of Nutrition* 3, No. 3 (1984).

6. Eric Braverman, et al., *The Healing Nutrients Within.* (Keats Publishing, Inc., 1997).

L.L. Rogers, "Glutamine in the Treatment of Alcoholism," *Quarterly Journal of Studies on Alcohol* 18, No. 4 (1957): 581–87.

L.L. Rogers and R.B. Pelton, "Effect of Glutamine on IQ Scores of Mentally Deficient Children," *Texas Reports on Biology and Medicine* 15, No. 1 (1957): 84–90.

Judy Schabert and Nancy Ehrlich, *The Ultimate Nutrient, Glutamine.* (Garden City Park, NY: Avery Publishing, 1994).

R.R.W.J. Van Der Hulst, et al., "Glutamine and Intestinal Immune Cells in Humans," *Journal of Parenteral and Enteral Nutrition* 21, No. 6 (1997): 310–15.

J. Li, et al., "Glutamine Prevents Parenteral Nutrition-Induced Increases in Intestinal Permeability," *Journal of Parenteral and Enteral Nutrition* 18 (1994): 3030–307.

J.C. Alverdy, "Effects of Glutamine-Supplemented Diets on Immunology of the Gut," *Journal of Parenteral and Enteral Nutrition* 14 (1980): 1095–1135.

M.I. Amores Sánchez and M.A. Medina, "Glutamine, as a Precursor of Glutathione, and Oxidative Stress," *Molecular Genetics and Metabolism* 67, No. 2 (June 1999): 100–05.

B.M. Lomaestro and M. Malone, "Glutathione in Health and Disease: Pharmacotherapeutic Issues," *Annals of Pharmacotherapy* 29 (1995): 1263–73.

R.F. Grimble, "Effect of Antioxidative Vitamins on Immune Function with Clinical Applications, Institute of Human Nutrition, University of Southampton, U.K.," *International Journal of Vitamin Nutrition Research* 67, No. 5 (1997): 312–20.

P. Furst, et al., "Glutamine Dipeptides in Clinical Nutrition," *Nutrition* 13, No. 7/8 (1997): 731–37.

H.G. Windmueller and A.E. Spaeth, "Identification of Ketone Bodies and Glutamine as the Major Respiratory Fuels in vivo for Post-Absorptive Rat Small Intestine," *Journal of Biological Chemistry* 253 (1978): 69–76.

Ziegler, et al., "Clinical and Metabolic Efficacy of Glutamine-Supplemented Parenteral Nutrition after Bone Marrow Transplantation," *Annals of Internal Medicine* 116 (1992): 821–28.

Hammarqvist, et al., "Addition of Glutamine to Total Parenteral Nutrition after Elective Abdominal Surgery Spares Free Glutamine in Muscle, Counteracts the Fall in Muscle Protein Synthesis and Improves Nitrogen Balance," *Annals of Surgery* 209 (1989): 455–61.

N.C. Jackson, et al., Department of Diabetes, Endocrinology and Metabolic Medicine, St. Thomas' Hospital, London, "The Metabolic Consequences of Critical Illness: Acute Effects in Glutamine and Protein Metabolism," *American Journal of Physiology* 276, No. 1 (January 1999): 163–70.

7. Billie J. Sahley, *GABA, The Anxiety Amino Acid*. (San Antonio, TX: Pain and Stress Publications, 1998).

   N.G. Bowery, et al., *GABA Receptors in Mammalian Function*. (New York: John Wiley and Sons, 1990).

8. Andre Barbeau and Ryan Huxtable, *Taurine*. (New York: Raven Press, 1975).

   Timothy Birdsall, "Therapeutic Applications of Taurine," *Alternative Medicine Review* 3, No. 2 (1998): 128–36.

   R.J. Huxtable and H. Pasantes-Morales, *Taurine in Nutrition and Neurology*. (New York: Plenum Press, 1981).

   R.J. Huxtable, "Physiological Actions of Taurine," *Physiology Review* 72: 101–03.

   Herminia Pasantes-Morales, et al., *Taurine: Functional Neurochemistry, Physiology, and Cardiology*. (New York: Wiley-Liss, 1990).

   Andre Barbeau and Ryan Huxtable. *Taurine and Neurological Disorders*. (New York: Raven Press, 1978).

9. Julia Ross, *The Diet Cure*. (New York: Penguin Group, 1999).

10. Julia Ross, *The Mood Cure*. (New York: Penguin Group, 2002).

11. Roger J. Williams, *Alcoholism: The Nutritional Approach*. (Austin, TX: University of Texas Press, 1959).

12. Kenneth Blum and Michael Trachtenberg, "Neurogenic Deficits Caused by Alcoholism: Restoration by SAAVE," *Journal of Psychoactive Drugs* 20 (1988): 297–312.

13. Raymond J. Brown, Kenneth Blum, and Michael Trachtenberg, "Neurodynamics of Relapse Prevention: A Neuronutrient Approach to Outpatient DUI Offenders," *Journal of Psychoactive Drugs* 22, No. 2 (April/June 1990).
14. Kenneth Blum, et al., "Neuronutrient Effects on Weight Loss in Carbohydrate Bingers: An Open Clinical Trial," *Current Therapeutic Research* 48 (1990): 217–33.
15. Billie Jay Sahley and Katherine M. Birkner, *Heal with Amino Acids and Nutrients*. (San Antonio, TX: Pain and Stress Publications, 2001).
16. Billie Jay Sahley and Katherine M. Birkner, *Heal with Amino Acids*. (San Antonio, TX: Pain and Stress Publications, 2001).

Chapter 6

1. B.A. Watkins, et al., "Food Lipids and Bone Health," in *Food Lipids and Health*, R.E. McDonald and D.B. Min, eds. (New York: Marcel Dekker, 1996), pp. 101–02.
2. G.H. Dahlen, et al., *Journal of Internal Medicine* 244(5) (November 1998): 417–24.
   P. Khosla and K.C. Hayes, *Journal of the American College of Nutrition* 15 (1966): 325–39.
   B.A. Clevidence, et al., *Arteriosclerosis, Thrombosis, and Vascular Biology* 17 (1997): 1657–61.
3. M.L. Garg, et al., *Federation of American Societies for Experimental Biology Journal* 2 (4) (1988): A852.
4. L.D. Lawson and F. Kummerow, *Lipids* 14 (1979): 501–03.
   M.L. Garg, *Lipids* 24(4) (April 1989): 334–39.
5. Presented by Sarah M. Conklin, Ph.D., Cardiovascular Behavioral Medicine Program, University of Pittsburgh, at the American Psychosomatic Society's Annual Meeting, Budapest, Hungary, March 2007.
6. For more information on the health benefits of coconut oil, see:
   A. Keys, A. Menotti, et al. "The Diet and 15-year Death Rate in the Seven Countries Study." *American Journal of Epidemiology* 124: 903–15 (1986).
   I.A. Prior, et al., "Cholesterol, Coconuts, and Diet on Polynesian Atolls: A Natural Experiment: The Pukapuka and Tokelau Island Studies," *American Journal of Clinical Nutrition* 34(8) (1981): 1552–61.

Bruce Fife, *The Healing Miracles of Coconut Oil*. (Colorado Springs, CO: Health Wise, 2001), 20–23.

Weston Price, *Nutrition and Physical Degeneration* (Keats Publishing, 1998).

W.C. Willett, "Diet and Coronary Heart Disease." *Monographs in Epidemiology and Biostatistics* 15: 341–79 (1990).

World Health Organization. "Diet, Nutrition, and the Prevention of Chronic Diseases. Report of a WHO Study Group." *WHO Technical Report Series* 797, Geneva, Switzerland, 1990.

Chapter 7

1. For more information on acupuncture, see:
   Manfred Porkert and Christian Ullman, *Chinese Medicine, Its History, Philosophy, and Practice*, translated and adapted by Mark Howson. (New York: William Morrow and Co., 1988).

2. Isadore Rosenfeld, *Dr. Rosenfeld's Guide to Alternative Medicine*. (New York: Random House, 1996).

3. For more information on Acu-Detox, see:
   Alex Brumbaugh, "Acupuncture: New Perspectives in Chemical Dependency Treatment," *Journal of Substance Abuse Treatment* 10, No. 1 (1993).
   Michael Smith, "Acupuncture and Natural Healing in Drug Detoxification," *American Journal of Acupuncture* 2, No. 7 (1979): 97–106.

4. For more information about Auriculotherapy, see:
   Jay M. Holder, et al., "Increasing Retention Rates Among the Chemically Dependent in Residential Treatment: Auriculotherapy and Subluxation-Based Chiropractic Care," *Molecular Psychiatry* 6, No. 1 (2001).
   Jay M. Holder, "Beating Addiction from Bondage to Freedom," *Alternative Medicine* (1999).
   Lisa Ann Williamson, "The Secret to Success: Auriculotherapy Treatment Helps Some with Addictions," *Staten Island Advance* (March 18, 2002).
   Kenneth Blum, et al., "Reward Deficiency Syndrome: A Biogenetic Model for the Diagnosis and Treatment of Impulsive, Addictive, and Compulsive Behaviors," *Journal of Psychoactive Drugs* 32, Supplement (November 2000): 55–57.

5. Hearing Before a Subcommittee of the Committee on Appropria-

tions, United States Senate, 103rd Congress, First Session, U.S. Government Printing Office.
R.B. Smith, "Cranial Electrotherapy Stimulation," in J.B. Myklebust, J.F. Cusik, A Samies, et al., *Neural Stimulation*, Vol. 2 (Boca Raton, Florida: CRC Press, Inc., 1983), 129–50.

6. Kristin Swartz and Eric Braverman, MD, "Cranial Electrotherapy Stimulation (CES)," *Townsend Letter for Doctors* (Dec. 1991). E. Braverman, R. Smith, et al. "Modification of P300 Amplitude and Other Electrophysiological Parameters of Drug Abuse by Cranial Electrical Stimulation," *Current Therapeutic Research* 48, No. 4 (October 1990); 586–96.

7. K.B. Smith, "Confirming Evidence of an Effective Treatment for Brain Dysfunction in Alcoholic Parents," *Journal of Nervous and Mental Disorders* 170, No. 5 (1982): 275–78.

8. E. Braverman, R. Smith, et al., "Modification of P300 Amplitude and Other Electrophysiological Parameters of Drug Abuse by Cranial Electrical Stimulation," *Current Therapeutic Research* 48, No. 4 (October 1990), 586–96.

9. E.K. Braverman, K. Blum, and K.J. Smayda, "A Commentary on Brain Mapping in 60 Substance Abusers: Can the Potential for Drug Abuse Be Predicted and Prevented by Treatment?" *Current Therapeutic Research* 48, No. 4 (1990): 569.

Chapter 8

1. M.B. Sterman, "EEG Biofeedback: Physiological Behavior Modification," Neuroscience and Biobehavioral Reviews 5, No. 3 (1981): 405–12.

2. Joel Lubar, et al., "Evaluation of the Effectiveness of EEG Neurofeedback Training for ADHD in a Clinical Setting, as Measured by Changes in T.O.V.A. Scores, Behavioral Ratings, and WISC-R Performance," *Biofeedback and Self-Regulation* 21, (1995): 83–99.

3. M.B. Sterman and L. Friar, "Suppression of Seizures in an Epileptic Following Sensorimotor EEG Feedback Training," *Clinical Neurophysiology* 33 (1972): 89–95. M.B. Sterman, et al., "Biofeedback Training of the Sensorimotor EEG Rhythm in Man: Effect on Epilepsy," *Epilepsia* 15 (1974): 395–416.

4. For more information about Beta Training Neurofeedback, see: V.J. Monastra, et al., "Assessing Attention Deficit/Hyperactivity

Disorder via Quantitative Electroencephalography: An Initial Validation Study," *Neuropsychology* 13 (1999): 424–33.
M.A. Tansey, "Righting the Rhythms of Reason: EEG Biofeedback Training as a Therapeutic Modality in a Clinical Office Setting," *Medical Psychotherapy* 3 (1990): 57–68.
5. *Colorado Springs Gazette*, April 29, 2004.
6. For more about the Alpha-Theta Protocol, see: E.G. Peniston and P.J. Kulkosky, "Alcoholic Personality and Alpha-Theta Brainwave Training," *Medical Psychotherapy* 4 (1991): 1–14.
7. Tony Stephenson, "Link Between Memory and Neurofeedback," *Imperial College London Reporter* 126 (February 5, 2003).

Chapter 10

1. Connie Higley and Alan Higley, *Reference Guide for Essential Oils.* (Olathe, KS: Abundant Health, 1998).
2. Isadore Rosenfeld, *Dr. Rosenfeld's Guide to Alternative Medicine.* (New York: Random House, 1996).

Chapter 11

1. Jack Trimpey, *The Small Book.* (New York: Dell Publishing, 1989).

Chapter 12

1. January 1996.
2. Regina Sara Ryan and John W. Travis, *The Wellness Workbook.* (Berkeley, CA: Ten Speed Press, 1981).
3. Diana W. Guthrie, *Alternative and Complementary Diabetes Care.* (New York: John Wiley and Sons, Inc., 2000).

Chapter 14

1. Matthew Fox, *The Coming of the Cosmic Christ.* (San Francisco Harper and Row, 1988): 32.
2. Larrene Hagaman, "Building the Temple Within," *The Restoration Witness* (September/October 1990): 4–12.

Suggested Reading

Amen, Daniel, *Healing ADD*. (New York: Putnam, 2001).

Beasley, Joseph D. and Susan Knightly, *Food for Recovery*. (New York: Crown Trade Paperbacks, 1994).

Blum, Kenneth and James Payne, *Alcohol and the Addictive Brain*. (New York: The Free Press, 1991).

Braly, James and Patrick Holford, *The H Factor Solution*. (North Bergen, NJ: Basic Health Publications, Inc., 2003).

Braly, James and Patrick Holford, *Hidden Food Allergies: The Essential Guide to Uncovering Hidden Food Allergies and Achieving Permanent Relief*. (Laguna Beach, CA: Basic Health Publications, Inc., 2006).

Braverman, Eric and Carl C. Pfeiffer, *The Healing Nutrients Within*. (New Canaan, CT: Keats Publishing, Inc., 1987).

Breggin, Peter, *Talking Back to Ritalin*. (Monroe, ME: Common Courage Press, 1998).

Breggin, Peter, *Toxic Psychiatry*. (New York: St. Martin's Press, 1990).

Cass, Hyla, *Eight Weeks to Vibrant Health*. (Columbus, OH: McGraw Hill, 2005).

Davis, Joel, *Endorphins: New Wave of Brain Chemistry*. (New York: The Dial Press, 1984).

DesMaisons, Kathleen, *Potatoes, Not Prozac*. (New York: Simon and Schuster, 1999).

Elkins, Rita, *Solving the Depression Puzzle*. (Pleasant Grove, UT: Woodland Publishing, 2001).

Gant, Charles and Greg Lewis, *End Your Addiction Now*. (New York: Warner Books, 2002).

Gant, Charles, *Alternative and Bionutritional Approaches to ADD and ADHD*. (Syracuse, NY: AFCO, 1997).

Gorski, Terence and Merlene Miller, *Staying Sober: A Guide for Relapse Prevention.* (Independence, MO: Herald House, 1986).

Guthrie, Diana, *Alternative and Complementary Diabetes Care.* (New York: John Wiley and Sons, 2000).

Higley, Connie and Alan Higley, *Reference Guide for Essential Oils.* (Olathe, KS: Abundant Health, 1998).

Ketcham, Katherine and William Asbury, *Beyond the Influence.* (New York: Bantam Books, 2000).

Mathews-Larson, Joan, *Seven Weeks to Sobriety.* (New York: Fawcett Columbine, 1997).

Miller, David and Kenneth Blum, *Overload: Attention Deficit Disorder and the Addictive Brain.* (Kansas City, MO: Andrews and McMeel, 1996).

Miller, Merlene, Terence T. Gorski, and David K. Miller, *Learning to Live Again.* (Independence, MO: Herald House, 1992).

Pert, Candace B., *Molecules of Emotion.* (New York: Scribner Publishing, 1997).

Reuben, Carolyn, *Cleansing the Body, Mind and Spirit.* (New York: Berkley Books, 1998).

Richardson, Wendy, *The Link Between ADD and Addiction.* (Colorado Springs, CO: Piñon Press, 1997).

Rosenfeld, Isadore, *Dr. Rosenfeld's Guide to Alternative Medicine.* (New York: Random House, 1996).

Ross, Julia, *The Diet Cure.* (New York: Viking, 1999).

Ross, Julia, *The Mood Cure.* (New York: Penguin Books, 2002).

Sahley, Billie and Katherine M. Birkner, *Heal with Amino Acids and Nutrients.* (San Antonio, TX: Pain and Stress Publications, 2001).

Weintraub, Skye, *Natural Treatments for ADD and Hyperactivity.* (Pleasant Grove, UT: Woodland Publishing, 1997).

Williams, Roger J., *The Wonderful World Within You.* (Wichita, KS: Biocommunications Press, 1998).

Young, D. Gary, *Aromatherapy: The Essential Beginning.* (Salt Lake City, UT: Essential Press Publishing, 1995).

Index

12-step programs. See treatment
  programs
12 Steps for Nutritious Eating, 127
5-hydroxytryptophan (5-HTP), 71,
  73, 82, 231

abstinence, 38–41; chronic symptoms, 58–62
Abstinence Symptom Severity Scale,
  98
acetylcholine, 139
acupressure, 134, 154, 222
acupuncture, 14, 15, 16, 131–33,
  136–37, 154, 163, 222, 223, 224;
  ear (auricular therapy or acu-
  detox), 135–37; needle-less. See
  auriculotherapy
addiction; behavioral, types of,
  41–44; causes and psychology of,
  19–47; consequences of dependence, 34–38; disease model,
  56–58; statistics on, 51–52
aggression, 22, 84
Alcoholics Anonymous (AA), 37,
  54–55, 56, 57, 124, 167–69
alcoholism, predisposition for. See
  addiction, predisposition for;
  warning signs. See addiction,
  warning signs and diagnosis
allergies. See food allergies
alpha-theta protocol, 147
amino acid therapy, 67–102
amino acids, deficiency, 67–70;

essential and nonessential, 69–70;
  forms of, 70; guidelines for choosing, 81, 88–90; related to addiction, 70–75, 77; scientific studies,
  78; side effects, 85–86
anemia, 122
anorexia, 44, 84
antibiotics, 121
antidepressants, 73, 84, 95–96, 231
antioxidants, 112–13, 115, 120, 126
anxiety, 17, 23, 25, 26, 29, 37, 53,
  59, 61, 62, 67, 72–74, 78, 96, 106,
  111, 126, 138, 139, 151, 174,
  176, 181, 182, 183, 197–201
aromatherapy. See essential oil
  therapy
art, benefits of, 195, 223
artificial sweeteners, 120
attention deficit hyperactivity disorder (ADHD), 14, 23, 29, 88, 139,
  143, 145–46, 171–72
auriculotherapy, 15, 135–37

balance, recovery and, 205–12
benzodiazepines, 95–96
beta training, 145–46
biofeedback (neurofeedback) 14, 15,
  16, 141–48
blood-brain barrier, 80
blood pressure, 62, 84, 141–42,
  149, 158, 164, 173–74, 176, 178,
  190, 193
blood sugar, 11, 62, 118, 120–21

Blum, Kenneth, 8, 14, 16, 76
body work, 149–55
brain, reward system, 21–25
brainwave biofeedback (neurofeedback), 141–48
brainwaves, 15, 138, 142, 143–46, 208
Braly, James, MD, 7, 16, 90, 98
Braverman, Eric, 139
breathing, deep, 176–77, 178
Bridging the Gaps, 98, 221–22
bulimia, 44
Burroughs, Stanley, 162

caffeine, 124, 126, 162, 179
calcium, 75, 122
cancer, 50, 70, 72, 84, 104, 108, 110, 180, 188
carbohydrates, 86, 105–07, 109, 110, 117–21, 122, 124, 125
Center for Education and Drug Abuse Research (CEDAR), 60
cerebrospinal fluid, 154
cholesterol, 75, 110, 117, 126, 190
Chronic Abstinence Symptom Severity Scale, 229
cigarettes. See smoking
Clown Chakra, 188
coaching, 171–72, 225
coconut oil, 114–17
cod liver oil. See DHA
coffee, 10–11, 124, 126, 127, 146
Community Addiction Recovery Association (CARA), 222–23
companions, animal. See pets
compassion, 215–16
concentration, poor, 22, 59–60, 73
consequences, addictive substance use, 34
counseling, 10, 16, 18, 52, 147, 153, 169–71, 214, 221, 224, 225, 226
Counseling and Mediation Services, 223

cranial electrical stimulation (CES), 138–39
craniosacral therapy, 154–55
cravings, alcohol and drug, 25, 26, 29, 58, 59, 61, 62, 67, 72, 73, 78, 79, 91, 97, 224, 226; carbohydrate, 22, 110, 118, 123, 124, 125
Cummings, Carol, 223

dairy products, 106, 107, 110, 122, 129
Dave's Buffalo Chili, recipe, 109
deep relaxation, 174–76
deficiency questionnaires, 231–34
delerium tremens (DTs), 95
denial, 64–65, 100
dependence, 35–36
depression, 14, 17, 22, 23, 44, 53, 59, 62, 67, 68, 73, 78, 84, 109, 111, 139, 143, 144, 145, 181
detoxification, 38, 45, 74, 93–97, 100, 147, 226
diabetes, 40, 50, 149, 180
dieting, extreme, 27, 44
disease model of addiction. See addiction, disease model
dopamine, 11, 22, 23, 24, 42, 68, 69, 71, 72, 73, 78, 82–85, 106, 138, 223, 224, 225
D-phenylalanine. See phenylalanine
drug hunger. See cravings, alcohol and drug
drugs. See medications
dynorphins. See opioid peptides
dysphoria, 53, 61

ear acupuncture. See auriculotherapy
earplugs, 191
eating disorders, 44, 84
education, 18, 97
eggs, 85, 106, 107, 109, 110, 122, 129
Ellis, Albert, 168
Emotional Freedom Technique, 222

endorphins. See opioid peptides
energy levels, 23, 38–39, 59, 72, 78, 106–07, 109
enkephalins. See opioid peptides
environmental toxins, 28
essential fatty acids (EFAs), 109–17
essential oil therapy, 157–64
Excel Treatment, 7, 224, 235
ExecuCare Addiction Recovery Center, 224
exercise, 58, 120, 125, 128, 142, 179, 180–84; aerobic, 183; stretching, 183–84
Exodus Treatment Center, 137

fatigue, 77, 118, 211
fats, 105, 108, 109–17, 119, 120, 121, 122
fiber, 105, 119, 120, 123
fish, 107, 108, 111
fish oil, 111–12
folate (folic acid), 84
food addiction. See eating disorders
food allergies, 27, 85
food and mood, 105–07
frequency ranges, brain, 143
fun, benefits of, 185–86

gambling, 41, 42, 43, 65, 73, 170
gaming addictions, 43
gamma-aminobutyric acid (GABA), 11, 22, 23, 24, 69, 70, 71, 74, 78, 86, 88, 89, 96, 225, 234
Gant, Dr. Charles, 7, 16, 23, 225
Gattefossé, René-Maurice, 158
genetics, as factor for addiction. See addiction, predisposition for
glutamine. See L-glutamine
glutathione, 68, 69, 71, 74, 84
glycemic load, 118–20
glycine, 68, 70, 71
goal setting, importance of, 171–72
guilt, 207, 211

hallucinations, 94
headaches, 133, 138, 159, 233
heart attack, 84
heart disease, 50, 62, 108, 110
Hitt, Dr. William, 224
Holder, Dr. Jay, 137, 139
homocysteine, 75, 84, 89
hormones, 62, 69, 73, 107, 131, 158
honesty, 64–65
human growth hormone, 69
hyperactivity, 14, 23, 73, 84, 145, 171
hyper-augmentation. See stimulus augmentation
hypertension, 73

immune deficiency, 84
infections, 84, 133
Inner Balance Health Center, 225
insomnia. See sleep disorders
insulin, 118, 121
intravenous nutritional therapy, 91–102
irritability, 10, 23, 62, 67, 73, 78, 88, 90, 94, 99, 118, 231

Joel Lubar and Associates, 144
joyful living, 212–13

Kenny G, 195
kidney problems, 74, 107
Krieger, Delores, 150
krill oil, 112–13
Kuntz, Dora, 150

laughter, benefits of, 185–86, 188, 191, 214
lauric acid, 116–17
L-cysteine, 68, 75. See also under amino acids
leaky gut syndrome, 74, 93
legumes, 118, 120, 121, 129
Levy, Dr. Thomas, 224
L-glutamine, 14, 71, 73–74, 78, 82,

85, 88, 89. See also under amino acids
libido, 78
Librium, 78
LifeStream Nutritional Consultation and Products, 225–26
liver problems, 50, 74
L-lysine, 123 See also under amino acids
long-chain fatty acids (LCFAs), 114–15
L-phenylalanine, 14, 68, 70–71, 72–73, 82, 88. See also under amino acids
L-tryptophan, 68, 71, 73, 80, 81, 82, 85, 86, 88, 89, 106–07, 118. See also under amino acids
L-tyrosine, 68, 71, 72, 73, 80, 88–89, 106, 179. See also under amino acids

magnesium, 75, 84, 89
malnutrition, addictive behavior and, 27
Manka, Debra, 225
marriage, effects of addiction on, 36
massage, therapeutic, 15, 149–50
Maultsby, Maxie, 168
meat, 85, 107, 108, 110, 111, 121–22, 129
Medaus Pharmacy, 226–27
medications, addiction to, 19; prescription to treat addiction, 16–17, 44–45, 52
meditation, 54, 55, 177, 178, 210, 211, 222, 225
Mediterranean diet, modified, 128
medium-chain fatty acids, (MCFAs), 114–15
melatonin, 71, 73, 83, 84
memory, enhancing, 113, 147–48, 178; problems with, 60–61, 62, 84; training, 147–48
methylcobalamin, 84

milk. See dairy products
minerals, 27, 68, 82, 83, 92, 103, 105, 118, 224, 226
monoamine oxidase inhibitors (MAOIs), 73
mood-altering substances, long-term use of, 28, 58
mood rings, 142
music, 11, 179, 185, 187, 192, 195, 223
mutual-help groups, 166–67
myofascial release, 152–53

NADH, 84
nausea, 90, 95
negative thinking, 41
nervous system, damage to, 13
neurofeedback. See brainwave biofeedback
neurotransmitters, 15, 21, 22–29
nicotine, 28, 31, 41, 50, 51, 97, 124, 232
noise sensitivity. See stimulus augmentation
norepinephrine, 22, 23, 68, 71, 72, 73, 82, 83, 84, 106, 138, 232
nutrient depletion, 58
nutrition, 62, 76, 78, 85, 86, 89, 103–29

obesity. See weight loss
obsessive compulsive disorder, 14, 26
olive oil, 113–14
omega-3 fatty acids, 111–12, 115, 116
opioid peptides, 22, 23, 24, 42, 62, 82, 132, 159, 178, 185
overeating. See food addiction

P300 brainwave, 139
pain, natural relief for, 23, 133, 149, 154; sensitivity (see stimulus augmentation)
panic attacks, 72, 234

paranoia, 23, 78
Parkinson's disease, 23
Peniston, Eugene, 147
pets, health benefits of, 190–91
phenylalanine, 14, 68, 70–71, 72–73, 82, 88, See also under amino acids
phenylketonuria (PKU), 73
play, benefits of, 185–86
positive thinking, 41, 200, 212
potassium, 75
potatoes, 119
poultry, 107, 108, 121, 129
prayer, 54–55, 202–03, 210–11, 223
prenatal conditions, 27
protein, 67, 69, 72, 74, 80, 88, 105, 106, 107–09, 121–22
pyroxidal-5-phosphate (P-5-P), 83

qi gong, 222

raindrop therapy, 161
Rational Recovery, 168
Recovery Systems, 76, 226, 235
reflexology, 135, 151, 162–63
Reiki, 150–51
relapse, 12–18, 40, 44, 51–53, 57–58, 71, 72, 76, 78, 90, 91, 93, 97, 100–01, 103, 104, 170, 173, 212–13, 221
relaxation, 22, 106–07, 143, 151, 154, 159, 174–75, 176–78, 179, 184, 194, 208, 222, 223
reward cascade, 24–25
reward deficiency, 25–33, 58, 83, 139
risk-taking behavior, compulsive, 41–44
Ritalin, 31
Rolfing, 152
Rosen, Martha, 153
Rosen method, 153–54
Rosenfeld, Dr. Isadore, 163
Ross, Julia, 7, 16, 76, 89, 90, 226, 235

S-adenosyl-methionine (SAMe), 84, 89
schizophrenia, 23
seizures, 79, 84, 95, 134, 143, 164
self-esteem, 77, 216, 217
self-medication, 13, 29–30, 40, 42, 62
serenity prayer, 202–03
serotonin, 11, 23, 24, 69, 71, 73, 78, 81–85, 106, 117–19, 138, 223
sex addiction, 41–42, 44
sexual abuse and addiction, 27
Shiatsu, 154
shoplifting, 42–43
Sisco, Tamea, 224
sleep, 179; disorders, 53, 59, 62, 105, 138, 143, 173; natural aids, 73, 84, 86, 88, 106, 111, 118, 159, 176–77, 179; REM, 179
smoking, 28
sobriety, stress of, 62–63
social drinking, 56
sodium, 75
soy, 111, 115
spiritual awakening, 13–14
sponsor, AA, 169
Sterman, Barry, 145
stimulus augmentation, 13, 14, 59, 61, 62, 75, 105, 191, 193, 195. See also under hypersensitivity
Stokes, Stanley, 221
stress, 10, 23, 26, 27, 53, 58, 59, 61, 62, 68, 70, 72, 75, 78, 85, 89, 97, 95, 110, 128, 131, 139, 142, 144, 149, 152, 165, 173–96, 197–203, 222–23
sugar, 41, 118, 120–21, 124. See also under carbohydrates
supplements, amino acid therapy support, 83–84
suicide, 17, 44, 49–50
Sutherland, William, 154

talk therapy, 223
taurine, 22, 69, 70, 74–75, 78, 82, 84, 86, 88, 89
tetrahydroisoquinoline (TIQ), 31, 32
therapeutic massage, 149–50
Therapeutic Touch, 150–51
thyroid hormone, 73, 116
tobacco, 28
tolerance, 30–33
touch, healing, 193
Tourette's syndrome, 14, 26, 143
tranquilizers, 73, 95–96, 106
trans-fatty acids (trans fats), 115
trauma, physical, 27
treatment programs, 57, 65, 93, 134, 221–27
trigger foods, 124–25
Trimpey, Jack, 168
tyrosine. See L-tyrosine

Upledger, John, 154

Valium, 95
vegetable oil, 111, 113, 115, 117, 161
vegetables, 106, 118, 120, 121–22, 123, 126, 129

vegetarians, 122
video games. See gaming addictions
violence, 22, 23, 73
Vita Flex Therapy, 162–64
vitamin A, 84
vitamin B, 72, 73, 80, 82, 83, 84, 89
vitamin C, 80, 89
vitamin E, 111
vitamins, 14–15, 27, 68, 88, 92, 93, 95, 97, 103, 105, 109, 118, 120, 122, 223, 224, 225
vomiting, 95

Walters, Dale, 143
water, 82, 105, 159, 161, 194
weight loss, 128, 180
Weil, Dr. Andrew, 176
whole grains, 118, 119, 123
wine, 104, 126
withdrawal symptoms, 13, 57, 58, 95, 134, 139, 224
work addiction, 43,

yoga, 150, 176, 177–78

zinc, 83, 84

About the Authors

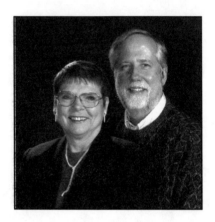

MERLENE AND DAVID MILLER are a husband and wife team
who have worked in the addiction field for twenty-five years
as authors, educators, consultants, and treatment professionals. They are relapse prevention specialists with a deep concern
for those for whom traditional treatment has not worked. The
Millers live in Missouri with their Papillion dog, Sammy.